KAUAI'S CHILDREN COME OF AGE

Kauai's Children Come of Age

Emmy E. Werner
Ruth S. Smith

The University Press of Hawaii / Honolulu

Manufactured in the United States of America

Library of Congress Cataloging in Publication Data

Werner, Emmy E   1929–
   Kauai's children come of age.

   Bibliography: p.
   Includes index.
   1. Child mental health—Longitudinal studies.
2. Psychology, Pathological. 3. Children in
Hawaii. I. Smith, Ruth S., 1923–   joint
author. II. Title.
RJ111.W47   362.7'8'20996941   76–56352
ISBN 0-8248-0475-9

To Jessie M. Bierman and Marjorie P. Honzik
with affection and admiration

Contents

Tables

Preface

Back in 1972, one of the candidates for mayor of Kauai, the "Garden Island" in the Hawaiian chain, ran his campaign on the slogan "Help Our Garden Grow." This catchy phrase was used throughout his term in respect to many basic economic, ecological, and even, occasionally, social needs.

About the same time, those of us who had been involved in the earlier research on the *Children of Kauai* (1971) began to plant some seeds in the appropriate bed—the Bureau of Community Health Services of the Department of Health, Education, and Welfare in Washington, D.C.—in the hope of germinating the necessary funds to learn how the human part of the garden had grown. This report is the result of that germination and much *hoe hana* (Hawaiian for "hard work in the fields") and tells the story of how a new generation came of age in the westernmost county of the United States.

We present here the findings from our follow-up in late adolescence of the children of Kauai, participants in a multidisciplinary longitudinal study that has lasted from the prenatal period to age 18. The unique aspect of this study was the opportunity to follow all pregnancies and births in an entire island community in Hawaii for nearly two decades.

In a previous book and in articles in professional journals, we have reported on the magnitude of reproductive and environmental casualties in this setting and on the short- and long-term effects of perinatal stress and a disadvantaged environment in early and middle childhood.

Thanks to the cooperation of nearly 90 percent of those who had participated at age 10, we have now been able to take a look at the learning disabilities and behavior disorders diagnosed in childhood, at new problems and new promises in adolescence, at the predictive power of our diagnostic tools, and at the community's response to its "youth at risk."

The 18-year follow-up was conducted under the joint auspices of the Community Services Council of Kauai and the University of California at Davis. This shared sponsorship allowed us to continue the constructive working relationship between professionals on both shores of the Pacific who had collaborated in the previous phase of the study.

Our deep appreciation goes to the educational, health, and social service agencies of the state of Hawaii who made it possible for us to conduct our research and allowed us the use of their facilities. In particular we extend our *mahalo* ("thanks") for gracious and extensive assistance to Barton H. Nagata, district superintendent, Department of Education, Kauai, to the office of Curriculum and Special Services, and to the staff of the three high schools on the island.

Our sincere thanks go also to the Department of Health, Divisions of Mental Health, Mental Retardation, and Public Health Nursing, to the Department of Social Services and Housing, Divisions of Public Welfare and Vocational Rehabilitation, to the Family Court, to the Kauai Police Department, and to Rehabilitation Unlimited Kauai, all of whom provided relevant data for our study.

In addition, we extend our appreciation to the G. N. Wilcox Memorial Hospital and Health Center and to the Kauai Veterans Memorial Hospital for their assistance in the conduct of our research and to the Kauai Community College for its cooperation.

We thank Sandra Machida Fricker, Sharon Howard, and Gail Kinnicut-Ryan for their unflagging efforts in data collection and we thank Keith Barton, Leanne Friedman, Linda Harnish, and Bidya Pradhan for their assistance in data analysis. Maude Hanohano and Laurie Smith were our local Girl Fridays in the initial and final phases of the project.

Financial support for the study came from the U.S. Public Health Service, Health Services and Mental Health Administration (Grant MC-R-060220-01/02-0), and from faculty research grants (1972–1974), University of California at Davis.

Our final aloha goes to the Chinese, Filipino, Haole (Anglo-Caucasian), Hawaiian, Japanese, Puerto Rican, and Portuguese youth of Kauai who cooperated so wholeheartedly with the study; to Earl, Myrna, Orville, and Stanley, who provided the moral support to see it through; and to Janis Castile, who patiently typed the manuscript.

CHAPTER 1
Introduction

From July 1972 to June 1974, two psychologists, one from the University of California at Davis and the other a clinical psychologist and resident of Kauai, conducted a follow-up study of a multiracial cohort of youth born on the island of Kauai, Hawaii, in 1955. Some 600 youth, approximately 90 percent of the original sample, participated.

The purpose of this report is to present the findings of this fourth phase of a longitudinal study that began in the perinatal period with an assessment of the reproductive histories and the physical and emotional status of the mothers from the fourth week of gestation to delivery. It continued with an evaluation of the cumulative effects of perinatal stress and quality of family environment on the physical, intellectual, and social development of the children at 2 and 10 years.

The Kauai study was unique in that it followed all births which occurred on the island—over a wide socioeconomic and ethnic spectrum—for nearly two decades. We gained a perspective on the magnitude of reproductive and environmental casualties in an entire community and on the cumulative effects of perinatal stress and a disadvantaged environment. We were also able to document the milieu and growth pattern of a substantial number of children from the lower end of the socioeconomic scale and from diverse cultural backgrounds. The results of our previous findings from the prenatal period to age 10 were published in *The Children of Kauai* (Werner, Bierman, and French, 1971). A brief summary of the major findings of our previous study can be found in Appendix 1.

The purposes of this report are to follow up where we left off at age 10, to document the course of the learning and behavior disorders diagnosed in childhood, to take a look at new problems and new promises in adolescence, to examine a concerned community's response to its youth at risk and factors that contributed to improvement, and to evaluate the predictive power of our diagnostic tools at birth, in infancy, and in childhood.

We hope that our findings will be of interest to policymakers and professionals who plan and deliver educational, social, and mental health services for the young and also to concerned citizens who care about the needs of a new generation coming of age.

In Chapters 1 to 3 we describe the objectives, the setting, and the population of our study and explain how we enlisted the cooperation of the community agencies and the youth of Kauai. We briefly review related studies on the long-term consequences of perinatal stress, learning disabilities, and childhood behavior disorders, contrast them with the design of our 18-year study, and delineate the three stages of our follow-up.

In Chapter 4 we discuss the long-term effects of moderate and severe perinatal stress on behavior in adolescence and contrast them with earlier findings at 2 and 10 years.

In Chapter 5 we present both the antecedents and the consequences of the learning disabilities diagnosed at age 10 and contrast their status at adolescence with that of a control group matched on relevant biological and environmental variables.

Chapters 6 and 7 review the outcomes of long- and short-term mental health problems diagnosed in childhood and contrast their status with that of youth without previous behavior problems.

Chapter 8 focuses on new problems which emerged in adolescence, especially delinquencies and teenage pregnancies, including abortions.

In Chapter 9 we illustrate the community's response to its youth with problems.

In Chapter 10 we compare youth whose status has improved with adolescents whose problems have persisted and discuss the contribution of treatment, family, and interpersonal variables to change in behavior.

In Chapter 11 we focus on subcultural differences in achievement orientation and socialization.

Chapter 12 is an overview of the 18-year status of the cohort of 1955 births, of the youths' plans for the future, and of their opinions on social issues of major concern to them: drugs, premarital sex, and race relations.

Chapter 13 examines the predictive power of our biological, psychological, and sociological "markers" in screening out potential problems in infancy, childhood, and adolescence.

In Chapter 14 we discuss the implications of our findings for developmental screening, early intervention, and legislation concerning children. We close with some thoughts on priorities for delivery of educational, mental health, and social services.

We hope that a discussion of both positive and negative outcomes, throughout this report, will help the clinically oriented reader to find a frame of reference for a meaningful interpretation of the general results that emerged from our statistical analysis.

Résumé of Longitudinal Studies

The report of the U.S. Joint Commission on the Mental Health of Children (1970) points to the urgent need for longitudinal studies that can yield information on such factors as the origins of disorders in human development, the continuity of such disorders throughout the life span, the factors that affect these disorders in both positive and negative directions over a period of time, and the timing and sequence of various behaviors.

To date, there has been only a handful of longitudinal studies that followed the course of normal child development through adolescence and into young adulthood. Descriptions of their goals, methods, and findings are summarized by Kagan (1964) and Sontag (1971). Seven longitudinal studies on the U.S. mainland have followed samples of (predominantly) Caucasian, (predominantly) middle-class children through the second decade of life:

1. On the West Coast: the Berkeley Growth Study (Macfarlane et al. 1954) and the Berkeley Guidance Study (Jones et al. 1971), both conducted by the University of California's Institute of Human Development

2. In the Midwest: the Nobles County study of the University

of Minnesota's Institute of Child Development (Anderson et al. 1959), the River City study of the University of Chicago's Committee on Human Development (Havighurst et al. 1962), and the Fels Institute Study at Yellow Spring, Ohio (Kagan and Moss 1962)

3. In the East: a study of temperament and behavior disorder (Thomas et al. 1968) at New York University and a follow-up of elementary school children in Brooklyn and Harlem into junior high school (Kraus 1973)

Only the Kauai study began as early as the *prenatal* period, followed *all* children in an entire community, representing *all* socioeconomic and ethnic groups on the island (predominantly Oriental and Polynesian), *and* maintained the cooperation of 90 percent of its sample throughout the second decade of life.

Three British studies have relevance to our own: a follow-up from birth to age 18 of a sample of 5,362 children born in a single week in 1946 in England, Wales, and Scotland (Douglas 1964); a population survey of all 10-year-olds residing on the Isle of Wight in 1964–1965, with a follow-up at age 14 (Rutter et al. 1970); and a survey of childhood behavior and mental health in a sample of 6,000 children, aged 5 to 15, in Buckinghamshire County, England, with a follow-up two to three years later (Shepherd et al. 1971). All these studies have been concerned with prediction over time, individual differences and their etiology, and individual developmental patterns among predominantly *normal* groups of children.

Follow-up Studies

LONG-TERM EFFECTS OF PERINATAL STRESS

Recent prospective studies of events occurring during pregnancy and the perinatal period and their associations with childhood disorders have focused on early and middle childhood. Only a few studies, notably the Collaborative Project (Berendes 1966; Broman et al.) and our Kauai study, have followed children at more than one time in their lives to observe both short- and long-term associations between perinatal complications and later development.

Some effects of perinatal stress may be minimal and transient; others may not show up until later in life. In the past decade, there have appeared a number of *retrospective* studies that have related low birthweight and prenatal and perinatal complications to later behavior disorders. Table 1 summarizes key findings from these studies.

Two previous follow-up studies of children who suffered from birth trauma and anoxia, one in France (Schachter 1950) and one in Chicago (Benaron et al. 1960), each covered a very wide age range (from 3 to 18 years) and included only a very small number of adolescents. Schachter included seven 18-year-olds among his 353 clinic cases and reported a greater incidence of emotional instability, truancy, cruelty, and theft among youth of puberty age who had suffered from birth trauma than among clinic cases of comparable age whose births had been normal.

Benaron et al. followed 41 anoxic children (predominantly black and from the lower socioeconomic class) at "some time" between 3 and 19 years. They noted a greater persistence of infantile habits as well as greater variability in IQ among anoxics than among (sib) controls. Some of the anoxic children showed superior intellectual ability, and the majority remained unaffected by severe birth complications.

Table 1 Retrospective Studies of Associations Between Reproductive Complications and Behavior Disorders in Childhood and Adolescence

Study	Low Birthweight	Prenatal Factors	Perinatal Factors
Schizophrenia in childhood and adolescence: with sib or twin controls			
Vorster (1960)		+	+
Taft and Goldfarb (1964)			+
Lane and Albee (1966)	+		
Pollack et al. (1969)			+
Stabenau and Pollin (1969)	+		+
Rutt and Offord (1971)			+
Schizophrenia in childhood and adolescence, psychotic, autistic, behavior disorders: with normal, unrelated controls			
Pasamanick and Knobloch (1960)	+	+	
Knobloch and Pasamanick (1962)		+	+
Hinton (1963)	+	+	
Zitrin et al. (1964)		+	+
Mednick and Schulsinger (1969)	+	+	+
Stott (1969)		+	

(+): Significant positive findings.

Mednick and Schulsinger (1969) studied a "high risk" sample of 20 Danish adolescents, born to schizophrenic mothers, who themselves manifested abnormal behavior by age 15. They found that the "sick" group had the largest number of birth complications: 53 percent of the "sick" group, 15 percent of the "well" group (other adolescents born to schizophrenic mothers who had not succumbed), and 28 percent of the normal controls (matched by age, sex, SES, and parental education) had severe complications, such as placental abnormalities, unfortunate fetal positions, unusually long labor, and mild prematurity (lower birthweight).

In sum: While there are hints from retrospective studies and three prospective studies with small samples of adolescents that severe perinatal stress may have some deleterious long-term effect on personality and social behavior, *no* longitudinal study has so far compared the short- vs. long-term effects of perinatal stress across the entire period from birth to the end of the second decade. This follow-up study at adolescence hopes to fill the gap.

LD / MBD CHILDREN INTO ADOLESCENCE

Wender (1971) has probably presented the most lucid discussion of the characteristics, etiology, prevalence, diagnosis, and prognosis of "minimal brain dysfunction" (MBD). The prevalence of the variant of the MBD syndrome most frequently seen—a hyperactive child of normal intelligence with a learning disability (LD), usually a reading or communication problem, and with impaired coordination of motor movements and visual-motor deficits—appears to range between 5 and 10 percent in the elementary school population (Stewart et al. 1966). In Kauai, we found hyperactive symptoms in 6 percent of the 10-year-olds, with a boy-girl ratio of 3:1. This agrees with findings of Paine, Werry, and Quay (1968) with Caucasian samples on the U.S. mainland. About 3 percent of our cohort had both hyperactivity and accompanying learning disabilities (22 out of 696).

On the basis of seven selected case studies of MBD children, Denhoff (1973) has recently charted some of the changing behavioral aspects of their natural life history as they move from infancy through childhood into adolescence: A highly reactive infant, with labile responses, becomes a toddler with exaggerated exploratory activity, a preschool child characterized by turbulent behavior, a hyperkinetic elementary school child with frustrations that emerge in poor academic achievement and low self-esteem by the time he or she reaches preadolescence. Recession in adolescence appears uneven and unpredictable.

In spite of the rash of current interest in these children by educators, pediatricians, psychologists, and child psychiatrists, controlled scientific follow-up data are sparse. Retrospective accounts have begun to appear in the medical literature, but there are only a handful of prospective studies that have followed MBD children into adolescence or adulthood. Attrition rates are high and, with the exception of one study which has published an interim report (Dykman et al. 1973), appropriate controls are lacking.

The results of recent follow-up studies are summarized in Table 2. The findings of all five follow-up studies reviewed here are rather discouraging and do not bear out the anecdotal evidence from parents and the helping professions that many of these children get appreciably better in adolescence.

There is little evidence for the assumption that the MBD child will "grow out" of his or her symptoms at the time of puberty—regardless of type of treatment (drug therapy, special education) or lack of it. Hyperactivity may disappear with adolescence, but other and perhaps more serious features of the syndrome may not. The MBD syndrome may be an early precursor of psychiatric and social conduct disorders, including serious academic underachievement.

The question of *which* MBD children develop in *what* ways, and the factors contributing to positive vs. negative outcomes, require further longitudinal research, such as the Kauai study, with proper controls and with attrition rates kept to a minimum.

CHILDHOOD BEHAVIOR PROBLEMS

About one child out of every six on Kauai at age 10 had behavior problems severe enough to interfere with school achievement; about 4 percent were considered in need of long-term (more than six months) mental health services as judged by an interdisciplinary panel consisting of a pediatrician, a clinical psychologist, and a public health nurse (French et al. 1968). Our findings agree closely with the prevalence rate for clinically significant psychiatric disorders reported for 10- and 11-year-old children in the Isle

Table 2 Follow-up Studies in Adolescence and Adulthood of the LD/MBD or "Hyperactive Child" Syndrome

Study	Age	Subjects	Findings*	
Weiss et al. (1971)	At diagnosis: 9 At follow-up: 13.3 Range: 10–18	64 of 155 MBD given drug therapy	Visual-motor skills Hyperactivity School achievement Self-concept Social behavior	O I P P P
Mendelson et al. (1971)	At diagnosis: 10 At follow-up: 13.4 Range: 12–16	83 of 140 hyperactive children given drug therapy and psychiatric counseling	Visual-motor skills Hyperactivity School achievement Self-concept Social behavior	O I P P P
Dykman et al. (1973)	At diagnosis: 10.5 At follow-up: 14.0	31 of 88 LD/MBD given special education; 22 controls	Visual-motor skills Hyperactivity School achievement Self-concept Social behavior	I I P P P
Laufer (1971)	At diagnosis: 8 At follow-up: 19.8 Range: 15–26	66 of 100 MBD given drug therapy	Visual-motor skills Hyperactivity School achievement Self-concept Social behavior	O I P O P
Menkes et al. (1967)	At diagnosis: 7 Range: 5–10 At follow-up: 22–40	14 of 18 selected with definite or probable MBD; no drug therapy	Visual-motor skills Hyperactivity School achievement Self-concept Social behavior	P I P O P

*O: Not studied.
I: Improvement.
P: Poor performance.

of Wight study in Great Britain (Rutter et al. 1970) and reported by Hagnell for children under 10 in Sweden (as quoted by Robins 1970:3–5).

The untreated emotionally disturbed child is expected to become eventually an emotionally disturbed adult, an axiom that Lewis (1965) has called the "continuity hypothesis." During the past decade a handful of follow-up studies have appeared in the literature that have checked this continuity hypothesis on populations of schoolchildren who had been screened for behavior problems in early elementary grades by using either teachers and peers or teachers and mothers as informants. The results of the follow-up studies on these children, some two to five years later, are summarized in Table 3.

Generally follow-up studies of populations of schoolchildren indicate a persistence rate of behavior problems that is *lower* than anticipated from follow-back studies of clinic populations. Only between 30 and 40 percent of the *same* children who had been screened in elementary school (usually in grades 1 to 5) reappear as persistent behavior problems in adolescence—even if no intervention has taken place in the time between first screening and follow-up. Unfortunately, the follow-up studies involving the largest number of children and reporting the lowest persistence rate suffer from a high attrition rate: 50 percent or more in the studies by the Onondaga County Schools (1964), Glavin (1972), and Kraus (1973). Thus we do not know how many of the persistent problem cases were missed. On the other side of the coin,

Table 3   Follow-up Studies in Adolescence of Schoolchildren Screened for Behavior Problems in Elementary Grades

Study	Number and Age of Subjects	Follow-up	Persistence of Problem	Attrition Rate
Onondaga County School Studies (1964): New York State	N=515 7–9 yr	2 yr later	31.3% (NT)	High (50%)
Stennett (1966): rural school district, northern Minn.	N=333 9–11 yr	3 yr later	40.0% (NT)	23%
Glavin (1972): Anderson County, Tenn.	N=773 7–11 yr	4 yr later	30% (NT)	High (54%)
Shepherd et al. (1971): Buckinghamshire, England	N=100 (50 T; 50 NT) 5–15 yr	2–3 yr later	39% (NT) 35% (T)	Low
Kraus (1973): black, white, Puerto Rican, Oriental subjects; Brooklyn and Harlem, N.Y.	N=165 5–9 yr	Up to 5 yr later	High*	High (50 %)

NT: Not treated.
T: Treated (parental guidance, psychiatric counseling).
* Actual percentage not given.

effective intervention should not only improve the problem child's subsequent adjustment, but ought also to effect a noticeable reduction in the future incidence of disorders. The evidence appears to contradict this "intervention hypothesis" as well.

A comprehensive review of 47 reports of the outcome of child psychotherapy, spanning a 35-year period, finds little support for the idea that treatment makes much difference (Levitt 1971). Improvement rates of two-thirds are regularly reported for *both treated and untreated* child populations studied, the control groups consisting of children subjected to the same diagnostic process as the treated cases, having been accepted for treatment, but having never received any formal therapy sessions (defectors).

The defector method has been criticized on the ground that defectors and treated cases are originally dissimilar on certain dimensions such as intensity of disturbance. One of the rare outcome studies that employed a true *random* sampling method, the Buckinghamshire County child survey in England (Shepherd et al. 1971), reports similar results as the studies which used defectors as controls (see Table 3).

The treated sample in the British study consisted of 50 randomly chosen "neurotic" children between the ages of 5 and 15, seen at child guidance clinics in the county over a period of two to three years, and a control group matched for age, sex, and symptoms, and selected from a random sample of more than 6,000 children in the county who had never obtained or sought psychiatric assistance. Outcome ratings were made by clinicians and based on interviews with parents. Sixty-five percent of the treated sample were rated as improved, as compared to 61 percent of the controls.

There were no differences between treated and untreated samples in severity of disturbance (as judged by number of "deviant" behavior symptoms), birth order, size of family, or easy access to clinic. The most obvious difference lay in the attitudes of mothers: Nonclinic children tended to have mothers who noticed that their children had problems but thought they were unavoidable; mothers of children who were referred to mental health clinics were more likely to feel worried about their children's problems. Parental attitude was also the key factor to improvement in both the treated and the untreated samples.

Childhood Predictors of Mental Health Problems

The best recent account of the current state of the art is Kohlberg et al.'s (1972) review of the predictability of adult mental health from childhood behavior. When we look at the results of the few longitudinal studies of (predominantly Caucasian) children that assessed achievement, emotional, and social problems in middle childhood and related them to later problems in adolescence and young adulthood, *low school achievement* and *antisocial behavior* emerge as the most powerful predictors.

One of the studies best controlling other factors (SES, IQ, race) and with a very low attrition rate is Robin's *Deviant Children Grown Up* (1966). This study followed the adult adjustment of 524 lower-class white children referred to a child guidance clinic in St. Louis in the 1920s and 1930s. Low school achievement did not differentiate children later becoming psychotic or neurotic from those who were well as adults, but it did predict later alcoholism, criminal, and sociopathic behavior. In an ongoing follow-up study of 235 black males who had attended St. Louis public elementary schools in the mid and late 1930s, Robins (1970) found that a combination of *truancy* (defined as absent 20 percent of time in five or more school quarters) and *being held back* (repeating two or more quarters or being placed in an ungraded room) *in elementary school* were powerful predictors of dropping out before high school (78 percent), diagnosable adulthood psychiatric disorders (66 percent), drug use (59 percent), and serious criminal records (57 percent).

Robins found little relationship between physical and emotional problems in childhood and probability of a maladjusted outcome in adulthood. There were no significant differences in childhood symptomatology between clinic cases who later became neurotic and those who were well as adults. The longitudinal evidence best documented by her study suggests, however, that antisocial behavior in middle childhood (i.e., aggressive, violent behavior, disobedience, poor relations with peers) is predictive not only of later criminal and sociopathic outcomes but of all other nonneurotic forms of maladjustment (i.e., alcoholism and psychoses). Antisocial behavior, particularly when some estimate of severity is taken into account, appears to be the single most powerful predictor of later mental health problems of any childhood behavior studied.

Some additional evidence on the predictive power of deviant behavior of a certain type and severity comes from three populations of normal school-age children followed longitudinally in the United States (in California, Minnesota, New York City) and one in England (the Buckinghamshire County survey).

Shepherd et al. (1971) in a British survey of childhood behavior and mental health found that *number* of items of deviant behavior (for ages 5 to 15 by sex) and *severity* of incapacitation were more predictive of later deviancy than attempts at classification by any one syndrome. Overall levels of symptoms on teachers' behavior ratings from grades 4 to 12 were also the best predictors of emotional disturbance and delinquency in the Nobles County study in Minnesota (Anderson et al. 1959; Werner and Gallistel 1961).

The Berkeley Guidance Study (Macfarlane et al. 1954) followed 116 children at yearly intervals from 21 months to 14 years. At each age, children were evaluated with regard to the presence or absence of 39 symptoms associated with biological and motor functions, social standards, and personality patterns. Most children's symptoms were age-specific. Exceptions to this rule were destructiveness, demanding attention, somberness, shyness, and excessive reserve. When these were present at age 6 or 7, they were also likely to be present in the same child at age 13 or 14. Although most specific symptoms changed from one age to another, children with many symptoms at one age tended to have many symptoms later on.

Certain temperamental characteristics may be predictive of later behavior disorders; Thomas et al. (1968) report that 70 percent of "difficult" infants (characterized by excessive activity, irritability, unpredictability, and high intensity) developed problems by age 9. In a later follow-up, Chess and Thomas (1969) note that children with irregularity in biological functions and distractible, irritable, highly active children had a much lower improvement rate (only 50 percent), when under treatment, than other age-mates diagnosed as having childhood behavior disorders (whose improvement rate reached 80 percent).

We conclude this brief résumé of related longitudinal

research with a comment by Kohlberg et al. in their report to the Joint Commission on the Mental Health of Children (1972:1271–1272):

> If the child clinical professions are ever to distinguish the children needing treatment from those who do not, it will depend on further longitudinal research. . . . Long-term effectiveness of treatment cannot be subject to research evaluation until we can isolate for treatment a group of children whose problems are predictive of later maladjustment and whom we can compare with a control group of children who we can also reliably predict will show an equal likelihood of later maladjustment. . . . From a practical point of view what is most urgently needed is a longitudinal evaluation of current methods and concepts of psychodiagnosis, including family interview and diagnostic tests.

While the studies reviewed here have focused primarily on Caucasian children from predominantly middle-class homes and had, with the exception of Robins (1966) and Shepherd et al. (1971), high attrition rates and limited time spans and controls, the Kauai study has been fortunate in being able to avoid some of these methodological shortcomings.

The Kauai study allows us to take a look at the effectiveness of current diagnostic tools and treatment modalities across a wide spectrum of children from different socioeconomic and ethnic groups, to examine the predictability of behavior from birth and infancy to adolescence, and to control for the effects of age, sex, IQ, SES, and ethnicity on "problem behavior" by careful matching from a large pool of participants whose attrition rate across two decades has remained remarkably low.

Here, then, are the objectives of our follow-up at age 17–18:

1. To assess the long-term consequences of the learning and behavior disorders diagnosed in childhood by age 10

2. To identify additional learning and behavior disorders that developed in the interval between 10 and 18 years

3. To evaluate the predictive validity of our diagnostic signs from our records at birth (including perinatal stress score) as well as psychological and pediatric examinations and family interviews at 2 and 10 years in forecasting later behavior and learning disorders

4. To examine the effectiveness of the community agencies' responses to youth at risk

5. To isolate demographic, family, and interpersonal variables that contribute to improvement in status

CHAPTER 2
The Community

Kauai, the "Garden Island" of the Hawaiian chain, has a very ancient name—*Kauai-a-mono-ka-lani-po*. Translated, this means "the fountainhead of many waters from on high and bubbling up from below." Although used in a different context in prior times, this phrase continues to be an apt reflection of the varying sources and forces contributing to present-day Kauai. The island's great natural beauty, encompassing mountains and cliffs, deep canyons and pounding surf, is considered to rank high among the earth's spectacular scenes. As the oldest of the Hawaiian islands, its history and legends reflect a certain maverick quality and independence of spirit which have come to characterize its people and their life-styles.

Settled in the eighth century A.D. or even earlier by canoe voyagers from the Marquesas and Society Islands, populated in the twelfth and thirteenth centuries by migrations from Tahiti, the Hawaiian Islands were rediscovered by Captain James Cook, England's great seagoing explorer, whose first landing occurred on Kauai in 1778. Christian missionaries from New England established the first mission in 1820; in 1835 the islands' first sugar plantation was founded in Koloa, on Kauai. The development of the plantations was the stimulus to the influx of what today constitutes Hawaii's polyglot population. Chinese, Portuguese, and Japanese were imported for plantation labor prior to the 1900s, with Puerto Ricans, Koreans, and Spaniards coming into Hawaii during the early twentieth century and large numbers of Filipino immigrants continuing to arrive until shortly after the end of World War II.

A Decade of Change

Kauai, lying at the northwest end of the Hawaiian chain, ranks fourth among the islands in geographical size and population. Containing 549 square miles of land, the population has grown from about 28,000 to 31,385 in the period during which our study's children have been growing up. While the early groups have largely assimilated, new immigrants, primarily from the Philippines and transient coast Haole (Caucasian) groups, have brought new attitudes and life-styles into the community.

Where Kauai's economy had once been based almost entirely on sugar and pineapple production, the period beginning with the late 1960s saw the development of the real boom in tourism which had started during the early years of our children. From 1966 to 1973 the agriculture labor force decreased from 2,230 to 1,680, all pineapple canneries closed down, and the tourism labor force increased from 1,850 to 2,700. Overnight visitors to Kauai rose from a total of 175,820 per year in 1966 to 590,475 per year in 1973. Sugar continues to be Kauai's major agricultural enterprise and will doubtless retain its primary position in the foreseeable future, but increasing consideration is being given to diversified agriculture. With increased mechanization, urbanization, and new local and export markets, the opportunities for Kauai's youth are shifting and the youngsters will find themselves forced to make decisions for the future based on the slight experience of their parents and themselves.

Other economic changes have been brought about by an increase in the government work force from 1,670 in 1966 to 2,220 in 1973. Since our study began, the space age has reached this remote island. Major scientific-military installations were developed on the west side of the island which have provided important contributions to the moon explorations and general strategic defense. They opened new possibilities to Kauai's people as well as introducing a new population to the island.

These economic and population shifts have had a significant effect on the young people. No longer willing to settle for the predictable futures of their fathers, but not necessarily prepared for other alternatives, some have left the island for Honolulu and the mainland. Others are experimenting with alternative life-styles or are involving themselves actively in the controversies surrounding these changes. Ecology groups such as Save Our Surf and Ohana O Mahaulepu have sprung up to resist the influx of developers and their efforts to change the environment by the addition of more hotels, condominiums, and a pace of life which the youth feel may destroy their heritage.

The advent of the so-called hippies, primarily from the West Coast of the mainland, at the time our cohort was entering its teen years added to the turbulence of this period. This group's search for serenity and inner awareness by the use of drugs, their desire for the simple life, and their rejection of established values brought social changes and conflicts totally outside the experience of our group. The harassment of one group by the other became a not uncommon occurrence. Although much misinformation exists on the extent and prevalence of drug abuse, all concerned agree that the problem has developed into a significant problem from a point of being virtually unknown when our youngsters were first studied. Drugs are now easily available, and youngsters have great freedom in deciding about their use.

Concurrent with this, the Police Annual Report of 1973 indicates a 50.12 rate per thousand of Pt. I offenses (murder, manslaughter, rape, robbery, burglary, theft) as compared to 19.0 per thousand in 1965 and an increase of motor vehicle accidents from 520 to 994. In this same period the number of police officers for the island has increased from 77 to 114.

Educational, Health, and Social Services

In an effort to cope with the many changes of the past decade, the educational and social agencies of the community have added new programs and shifted their focus and *modus operandi*. Private groups have increased their services as well and formed their own committees for further study.

Kauai still has three high schools, but in addition to the special classes for the mentally retarded, many programs have been added—programs for potential dropouts, work motivation classes, special classes and programs for pregnant teenagers, Outreach counselors, and special off-campus classrooms. The

Special Services offices maintain a staff consisting of a coordinator, two psychological examiners, two speech and hearing specialists, social workers, and visiting teachers as well as diagnostic-prescriptive teachers.

The growth of our cohort saw also the early growth and expansion of the Kauai Community College. Starting with a student enrollment of about 250 in 1965, the college in 1973 served a thousand students. The projected enrollment for this branch of the University of Hawaii is 1,500 students.

Partly as a result of the findings reported in *Children of Kauai*, the State Health Department on Kauai formed the Kauai Children's Services, a coordinated multidisciplinary and one-door entry approach to its services for children—services related to child development, developmental disability, learning disability, mental health, mental retardation, pediatrics, orthopedics, cardiology, and other special fields. Specialists from Honolulu together with local public health nurses, physicians, social workers, and psychologists are available for diagnostic and treatment services. The Kauai Community Mental Health Service has a staff of two psychiatrists, a clinical psychologist, two social workers, and two paramedical assistants. Its treatment emphasis has shifted to crisis intervention and the "systems approach." As this report was completed, the state legislature had just funded special children's mental health teams to be attached to each of the state's cachement areas. Kauai could anticipate the services of four additional mental health professionals to work with its youth.

Medical services have greatly accelerated during this period. Where 1966 saw one physician for every 4,800 persons, 1972 figures show one per 990 people, with a total of 36 physicians in practice at the conclusion of our data collection in 1974. Probably the greatest contribution to medicine in the past four years has been the recruitment of medical specialists—from one board- certified practitioner to the coverage of 22 basic specialties. Three hospitals continue to serve the population, but a greater level of care is noted, including family planning and implementation of the liberalized abortion laws.

Social agencies likewise have expanded staff and services. The Family Court and the Department of Social Services and Housing's Divisions of Public Welfare and Vocational Rehabilitation all maintain extensive case loads, and their staffs participate actively in community planning. The Police Department has increased its services to provide a special female counselor in its Juvenile Crime Prevention Unit and a school relations officer at one of the high schools.

Rehabilitation Unlimited Kauai, with its vocational evaluation and training programs and sheltered workshop, provides one of the island's major resources for both youth and adults. Kauai Economic Opportunity, Inc., and Headstart have developed programs to assist residents of all ages in target areas to deal with their problems and improve their quality of life, while the Commissions on Children and Youth and Aging promote studies of and activities for the juniors and the seniors in the island's population.

Kauai Community Services Council through its sponsorship of such programs as the Committee on Substance Abuse, the Kauai Immigration Services Committee, the Serenity House (a halfway house for recovering alcoholics), and its role as a coordinating and educational body for community services has broadened the base of service operations.

The Big Brothers and Big Sisters Association of Kauai, a nongovernmental organization, was formed and flourished during our youngsters' teen years. Other voluntary organizations such as the YWCA, YMCA, Civil Air Patrol, Catholic Youth Organization, Boy and Girl Scouts, and athletic groups provide recreational and learning experiences. During the latter part of this study efforts were being made by concerned members of the community to establish a residential group facility for children. Hale Opio Kauai (Youth Home of Kauai) opened its doors in July 1975. Its focus is on counseling, remedial education, development of prevocational skills and coping abilities, and the major goal of returning children to their families and the community as better-integrated persons.

This, then, is how the community appeared as we began our follow-up in late adolescence. One wonders if any other generation among Kauai's children had been exposed to so many and such rapid changes.

CHAPTER 3
Methodology

The general design of our follow-up study at ages 17–18 focused on (1) a survey of the entire cohort of 1955 births on the island of Kauai via a search of educational, health, and social service agency records, group tests of ability, achievement, and personality, and a biographical questionnaire and (2) an in-depth study via interviews of selected groups of youth at risk and control youth, without problems, matched by age, sex, socioeconomic status, and ethnicity.

The Sample

In Table 4 we present some relevant demographic data on the entire population of 1955 births on Kauai and subsamples of youth at risk and controls. In this table ethnicity is based on a cultural definition and refers to the country of origin of the child's immigrant ancestors—i.e., whether they were Chinese, Japanese, Filipino, Puerto Rican, or Portuguese (Lind 1955, 1967). It has remained a custom in Hawaii to designate Caucasians of North European or American ancestry as Haole ("stranger"). A person of any Hawaiian ancestry, no matter how slight the admixture of native blood, if it is recognized and known, is designated as part-Hawaiian. Since 1950, part-Hawaiians have been included with pure Hawaiians in most census tables. Other ethnic mixtures include children of two different non-Caucasian and non-Hawaiian parents; on Kauai they are mostly children of younger Japanese mothers and older Filipino fathers. All ethnic groups, of course, share in a common local "island culture." Socioeconomic status ratings are based on the father's occupation, income level, steadiness of employment, and condition of housing. The rating is based primarily on father's occupation, categorized by one of five groups: (1) professional; (2) semiprofessional, proprietorial, and managerial; (3) skilled trade and technical; (4) semiskilled; and (5) day laborer and unskilled. The majority of the youth are of Oriental and Polynesian descent (Japanese, Filipino, Hawaiian and part-Hawaiian) and more than half come from poor families.

The Cooperating Agencies

We were very fortunate to have the backing of an unusually helpful island community which had taken considerable pride in this study and had initiated several community action and compensatory education programs on the basis of our findings at ages 2 and 10 years.

It should be noted here that it had been agreed at the end of the 10-year follow-up that the general findings, including those of significance for individual children needing help, would be made available to everyone concerned. Letters with suggestions for follow-up and referrals to special agencies, where indicated, went to the parents, and reports of special diagnostic examinations went to the child's physician. With parental consent, reports were also sent to the Department of Education's Office of Guidance and Special Services and the Division of Mental Health of the local Department of Health if the parent initiated a follow-up contact. The psychologist gave several reports on the educational and mental health needs of problem children identified in the study at age 10.

Thus in comparison with previous phases of this longitudinal study, much of the need for publicity and acquainting the community with the purpose of the follow-up at age 18 was lessened. We were also extremely fortunate to have the sponsorship of the Community Services Council of Kauai, an umbrella organization of all educational, health, and social service agencies in the community, and to be able to tie some of our data collection into the ongoing program of the three high schools on the island.

We used multiple criteria to assess the status of the youth in

Table 4 Demographic Characteristics of 1955 Cohort and Subsamples of Youth at Risk and Controls

Characteristic	Percentage of 1955 Cohort (N=698)	LMH (%) (N=25)	LMH-C (%) (N=25)	SMH (%) (N=60)	SMH-C (%) (N=60)	LD (%) (N=22)	LD-C (%) (N=22)	NP (%) (N=45)
Sex								
Male	50	56	56	50	50	64	64	33
Female	50	44	44	50	50	36	36	67
Ethnicity								
Japanese	33	16	16	14	14	18	18	15
Filipino	18	24	24	24	24	18	18	22
Hawaiian and part-Hawaiian	22	16	16	25	25	36	36	43
Other ethnic mixtures	14	36	36	17	17	14	14	13
Portuguese	6	4	4	12	12	9	9	5
Puerto Rican	1	0	0	5	5	0	0	0
Chinese	1	0	0	0	0	4	4	0
Anglo-Saxon (Haole)	3	4	4	2	2	0	0	0
Socioeconomic status								
Very high (1)	2	0	0	0	0	0	0	0
High (2)	7	0	0	5	5	5	4	4
Middle (3)	35	12	12	24	24	18	18	21
Low (4)	42	56	64	50	66	50	50	50
Very low (5)	14	32	24	21	5	27	28	25

LMH: Long-term mental health problems.
SMH: Short-term mental health problems.
LD: Learning disabilities.
NP: New problems.
C: Controls.

the 1955 cohort in late adolescence. Records of contacts with agencies throughout adolescence, group tests of ability and achievement routinely administered in the local high schools in grades 8, 10, and 12, personality tests, interviews with the problem youth and closely matched controls in the senior year—all provided independent checks on the validity of our findings.

The Three Stages of the Follow-up

STAGE I: THE RECORD SEARCH

During our previous follow-up studies at ages 2 and 10, we had been impressed by the amount of useful information that was available on the children in the educational, health, and social service records of the community agencies on the island. We obtained permission to examine the records of the following agencies for data on referral (date, source, and reason), diagnosis, type of services rendered, and outcome, for the period between the end of our last follow-up and the present (1966 to 1973):

1. Department of Education, Office of Guidance and Special Services: records of periodic evaluations of all children placed in special classes for the mentally retarded, in learning disability classes, in special motivation classes for potential dropouts; records of special services for behavior, health, and learning problems

2. Department of Health, Divisions of Mental Health, Mental Retardation, and Public Health Nursing: records of all youth referred to community mental health services as outpatients or admitted to psychiatric hospitals; records of all youth with significant health problems, including the mentally retarded, and boys and girls served through Crippled Children's Services and the Public Health Nursing Branch

3. Department of Social Services and Housing, Division of Vocational Rehabilitation: records of youth who were physically disabled or slow learners and who were placed in work-study or Job Corps programs

4. Department of Social Services and Housing, Division of Public Welfare: records of all youth eligible for welfare benefits and families eligible for Aid to Dependent Children (ADC); foster home placements; home visits of social workers to families "in trouble"

5. Family Court and Kauai Police Department: records of

contact with law enforcement agencies, delinquent acts (including possession and sale of drugs); placement on probation, in Hawaii youth correctional facilities, or investigatory status; suicide attempts

6. Rehabilitation Unlimited Kauai: records of severely retarded and multiply handicapped youth who work in sheltered workshops and are participating in prevocational evaluation and training programs

7. G. N. Wilcox Memorial Hospital and Health Center and Kauai Veterans Memorial Hospital: records of teenage deliveries and abortions among the women in the cohort of 1955 births (checked by a professional records consultant)

A similar search was made of the Department of Education (Special Services), Department of Social Services, and Family Court records in Honolulu and on the other islands to which some youth from the 1955 cohort had moved.

STAGE 2: GROUP TESTS AND QUESTIONNAIRES

Tests of Ability and Achievement. The district superintendent, Department of Education, Kauai, gave us permission to copy from the records of the Special Services Division the following scores from group ability and achievement tests that had been routinely administered in grades 8, 10, and 12 in the high schools on the island: midpercentile scores on the verbal, quantitative, and total scales of the Cooperative School and College Ability Tests (SCAT 1966) and midpercentile scores on the reading, writing, and mathematics scales of the Sequential Tests of Educational Progress (STEP 1966).

Personality Tests. The California Psychological Inventory (CPI) (Gough 1969) and the Novicki Locus of Control Scale (Novicki and Duke 1972) were administered in group sessions to members of the 1955 cohort still attending high schools on the island. Follow-up sessions were scheduled for youth who could not be reached in the first round of testing. Youth at risk were given the group tests at the time of the interview if they had not participated previously in a group testing session.

Both the CPI and the Locus of Control Scale are well established, highly reliable, and widely validated instruments that have been used in longitudinal research (Block 1971; Havighurst et al. 1962) with samples of Caucasian youth in late adolescence and in cross-cultural research with Japanese and Hawaiian secondary school students (Brislin et al. 1973; Novicki and Duke 1972). Brislin et al. in their 1973 book *Cross-Cultural Research Methods* list both the CPI and the Locus of Control Scale as cross-culturally appropriate psychological tests. Thus our findings with Kauai youth can be meaningfully linked to other longitudinal and cross-cultural research.

The 18 CPI subscales cluster in four classes: (1) measures of poise, ascendency, self-assurance, and interpersonal adequacy; (2) measures of socialization, maturity, responsibility, and interpersonal structuring of values; (3) measures of achievement potential and intellectual efficiency; and (4) measures of intellectual and interest modes.

The Novicki Locus of Control Scale (I-E scale) measures the degree to which a person believes that a behavioral event is contingent upon her or his own action. Those who believe that events happen to them as a result of fate, luck, and other factors beyond their control are called "externals"; "internals" believe that their own actions determine the positive or negative reinforcement they receive. The Locus of Control Scale has stimulated a great deal of research, some of it cross-cultural. In all the reported ethnic studies, groups without power, either by virtue of social class or race, tend to score higher in the external control direction. Within the racial groupings, class appears to interact, so that the double handicap of lower class and lower caste seems to produce persons with the highest expectancy of external control. Brislin et al. have recently pointed out (1973) that the concept of internal-external control is not so unitary as was once hoped it might be. A variety of conditions and measures can alter the dimensions it seems to tap. Nevertheless, the concept of control from "within" or from "not within" is a fetching one for cross-cultural research.

Biographical Questionnaire. A brief biographical questionnaire (see Appendix 4) asking for information on educational status and plans, vocational status and plans, and marriage and health status was mailed to members of the 1955 cohort in a self-addressed and stamped return envelope. For youth at risk and controls this information was obtained during the course of the interview.

STAGE 3: INTERVIEWS

The following groups of youth at risk were selected from the cohort of 1955 births for an in-depth study via interviews:

1. All youth who had been diagnosed as LD at age 10 and for whom placement in a special learning disability class had been recommended by a panel consisting of a pediatrician, a psychologist, and a public health nurse (LD = 22).

2. All youth who had been diagnosed as being in need of long-term mental health services (more than six months) (LMH = 25).

3. All youth who had been diagnosed as being in need of short-term mental health services by the same panel at age 10 (SMH = 60).

4. New behavior problems that had arisen in the interval between the 10 and 17–18 year follow-up and were still persisting in late adolescence (NP = 45). They included prolonged truancies and dropouts, serious delinquencies (including drug abuse), illegitimate teenage pregnancies and abortions, suicide attempts and youth who had been admitted to psychiatric hospitals or referred to local mental health services. Detailed descriptions of the characteristics of the new problems are given in Chapter 8.

5. Control groups of youth, matched with the learning disability (LD-C) and long-term mental health cases (LMH-C) by age, sex, SES, and ethnicity, who had *no* learning or behavior problems at ages 10 or 18. Originally we had also planned to interview control groups of youth matched on the same criteria with the short-term mental health cases. Time did not permit this, but in our data analysis we will contrast all *other* 18-year follow-up data (i.e., agency contacts, ability, achievement, and personality test results, ratings of the family environment, and our findings at birth and ages 1, 2, and 10 years for the short-term mental health cases) with controls (SMH-C) drawn randomly from our 1955 cohort who are matched by sex, SES, and ethnicity. The distribution of problem and control groups on the criteria for matching (sex, SES, ethnicity) is given in Table 4.

A detailed description of the criteria used to diagnose children in groups 1, 2, and 3 above can be found in Chapters 5, 6, and 7 respectively.

The interviews (average length one to two hours) were concerned with the youths' overall attitude toward school, their achievement motivation, the realism of their educational and vocational plans beyond high school, and the extent of their participation in social activities and quality of social life. Also covered were their identification with their mother and father, their feelings of security as part of their family, the extent of their goal and value differentiation and self-insight, and the intensity of their conflict feelings and their self-esteem. A copy of the interview questions and ratings can be found in Appendix 4. The ratings allow for a comparison between the findings of the Kauai study and other longitudinal studies of Caucasian youth on the mainland, among them a longitudinal study of the mental health of rural youth in Minnesota (Anderson et al. 1959) and the intergenerational studies of the University of California's Institute of Human Development (Jones et al. 1971), still in progress.

Every effort was made to trace all youth at risk and the controls, including those who had moved to other islands in the state of Hawaii (mostly Honolulu, Oahu) and the mainland (mostly California). Ninety percent of the interviews were conducted by the resident psychologist on Kauai, the others by the project director in California and two graduate students in Honolulu. Reliability of interview ratings (made independently of any knowledge of other follow-up data was highly satisfactory and ranged from the high nineties to the high eighties (see Table 49 in Appendix 4).

The interviews extended over a one-year period from spring 1973 to spring 1974. During the few remaining months of the academic year 1972–1973 during which early 1955 births were still in grade 12, arrangements were made to interview them at the local high schools. Following graduation or withdrawal from high school, appointments were made to meet them in their homes, at the Department of Health centers on the island, in local libraries, and for those continuing their education, at the campuses of Kauai Community College, the Honolulu and Hilo campuses of the University of Hawaii, and university campuses in California. During the academic year 1973–1974 the late 1955 births who were still in grade 12 were again interviewed in the local high schools.

Contacting out-of-school youth in the community was difficult since many had full-time jobs or were less accessible to the interviewers, such as the teenage mothers with small children.

Up to three or four repeat appointments were scheduled if youth, usually those with problems, did not keep their first date. All participants who could be reached were contacted in person. If repeated attempts to establish contact were fruitless or, in the case of those who had joined the armed forces or were living beyond the traveling range of the staff on the U.S. mainland, impossible, the interview was mailed to the youth with an explanatory letter, a self-addressed and stamped return envelope, and an offer of $5 for completing the accompanying form. Less than 5 percent of the interviews were obtained in this manner.

In Table 5 we summarize the follow-up data obtained at 17–18 years from the three stages of our follow-up. As can be seen, we were able to obtain some 18-year follow-up data on 614 youth (88 percent of the 1955 cohort on whom we had 2- and 10-year data) and interview data on between 82 and 91 percent of the youth at risk. This represents a relatively low rate of attrition for a longitudinal study involving many persons over nearly two decades. By comparison, the two largest follow-up studies on the U.S. mainland, the Berkeley Growth Study and the Berkeley Guidance Study (Block 1971) and the St. Louis study of former child guidance clinic cases by Robins (1966), were able to reach 70 percent and 82 percent of their original target groups respectively.

The promise of a relatively stable sample on the island of Kauai remained justified across two decades of very rapid social change. At the time of the two-year follow-up, 96 percent of the living children were still on Kauai and available for study; eight years later, at the ten-year follow-up, we were able to locate 90 percent. The relatively small attrition rate in the remaining eight years is a tribute to the cooperation of an immensely helpful island community—to the education, health, and social agencies, to the parents, and especially to the youth themselves.

Strategies for Data Analysis

In the chapters to follow we present the differences obtained by chi square, Fisher's exact probability tests, and t tests between the youth at risk and their controls on the agency records, interviews, ability, achievement, and personality tests at age 18, and selected variables from birth, age 1, age 2, and age 10. We used two-way analysis of variance (ANOVA) tests to examine ethnic and socioeconomic differences on ability and achievement tests in our

Table 5   17–18-Year Follow-up Data on 1955 Cohort

Data	Number (N=698)	Percentage of Cohort
Deaths between 10 and 18 years	2	
Those for whom 17–18-year follow-up data are available	614	88
Biographical data (education, vocation, marriage, health)	560	80
SCAT (grades 8, 10, 12)	498	72
STEP (grades 8, 10, 12)	497	71
Novicki Locus of Control Scale	407	58
California Psychological Inventory	378	54
Agency records	293	42
Police	128	23
Public Welfare	94	14
High school counselors and principals (grade 12)	61	9
Special Services, Department of Education	55	8
Public Health Nursing and Mental Retardation	51	7
Family Court	48	7
Mental Health	30	4
Kauai hospitals: teenage pregnancies (deliveries and abortions)	28	8*
Vocational Rehabilitation and Rehabilitation Unlimited Kauai	14	2
Interviews with youth at risk and matched controls		
SMH problems at 10	49/60	82
LMH problems at 10	21/25	84
Controls for LMH	21	
LD at 10	20/22	90
Controls for LD	20	
New problems	41/45	91

* Percentage of females.

total 1955 cohort and discriminant function analysis to evaluate differences between the ethnic groups, by sex, on the subscales of the California Psychological Inventory. Finally, multiple regression techniques were used to test, step by step, the predictive power of our biological, psychological, and sociological markers in screening out potential problems in early and middle childhood as well as in late adolescence.

In the chapters to follow, we present selected case studies and relevant vignettes from individual interviews to illustrate both positive and negative outcomes among our youth at risk—youth who suffered moderate to severe perinatal stress, youth in need of learning disability classes, youth in need of long- and short-term mental health services, and youth with new problems in adolescence, foremost the delinquents and teenage pregnancies. We hope thus to present an effective balance between, on the one hand, the statistical findings that depict group trends and, on the other, individual life histories that illustrate stability and change in human behavior and the resiliency of youth.

CHAPTER 4
Perinatal Stress

In the early years of this longitudinal study, each child was given a clinical rating based on the presence of conditions thought to have a deleterious effect on the fetus or newborn. This evaluation was made by a pediatrician who scored the severity of some 60 complications or events which could occur during the prenatal, labor, delivery, and neonatal periods and then assigned an overall rating: 0, not present; 1, mild; 2, moderate; 3, severe. A summary of the scoring system for prenatal and perinatal complications is presented in Appendix 2. Among the survivors in the 1955 cohort, 30 percent suffered mild (1); 10 percent, moderate (2); and 2 percent severe (3) perinatal stress.

Effects by Age 2

At age 2, we found a direct relationship between severity of perinatal stress and the proportion of children rated below normal in physical status by the pediatricians who examined them. Whereas 11 percent of the children without perinatal complications were considered to be below normal in physical status, 23 percent of the children with moderate perinatal stress and 36 percent of those with severe stress were classified in this category. The latter had major congenital defects requiring long-term specialized medical care.

Retardation in cognitive development was especially pronounced for children with moderate to severe perinatal complications: On the basis of *both* test performance (Cattell Infant Intelligence Scale) and observations of the child's behavior, the psychologists independently rated 29 percent of the children with severe perinatal complications below normal and another 29 percent questionable. Of those with moderate perinatal complications, 22 percent were considered to be below normal and 12 percent questionable. However, the effects of perinatal stress on intellectual status at age 2 appeared to be greater among children whose parents were poor, had little education, or were unstable than among children whose parents were better off economically, better educated, and more stable.

Even before the children had reached their second birthday, Cattell IQ differences between children with severe perinatal stress growing up in a favorable early home environment and those with stress growing up in poverty were much larger (34 IQ points) than differences between children *with* and *without* perinatal stress growing up in a middle-class, stable home where parents had completed high school (7 IQ points).

Effects by Age 10

By age 10, differences found between children with various degrees of perinatal complications and those without perinatal stress were less pronounced than at age 2 and centered on a small group of survivors of severe perinatal stress. The greatest effects of perinatal complications were found in the proportion of children who required placement in special classes or institutions, had IQs below 85 (in the slow learner and mentally retarded categories), and had significant physical problems (predominantly defects of the central nervous system and musculoskeletal system and problems with vision, hearing, and speech). Among the mentally retarded at age 10, for instance, the incidence of moderate perinatal stress was twice as high as in the total 1955 cohort; the incidence of severe stress was 10 times as high.

The effect of the family environment was even more powerful than was apparent at age 2 and accounted for more of the variance in IQ than did degree of perinatal stress.

Among the youth at risk who are the subjects of our 18-year follow-up, children considered in need of long-term mental health services at age 10 had twice as high an incidence of *moderate* perinatal stress (16 percent) as controls matched by age, sex, SES, and ethnicity and twice as high an incidence of *severe* perinatal stress as the total 1955 cohort (4 percent).

Among children considered in need of short-term mental health services at age 10, the incidence of moderate perinatal stress did not differ from that of the population of 1955 births nor from controls matched by age, sex, SES, and ethnicity, but the incidence of *severe* perinatal stress (5 percent) was more than twice that in the total cohort.

There were no youngsters who had suffered from severe perinatal stress among those for whom placement in learning disability classes had been recommended at age 10, but the incidence of *moderate* perinatal stress in this group was higher than that for controls matched by age, sex, SES, and ethnicity. However, because of the small number of subjects in these groups, results of chi-square tests did not reach a statistically significant level.

Effects by Age 18

As can be seen from Table 6, four out of five of the youth who had suffered *severe* perinatal stress at birth still had significant behavior, learning, and physical problems in late adolescence. Nearly one-third were classified as mentally retarded (29 percent); one-fifth had become delinquent, among them many repeaters (21 percent); and 15 percent had significant mental health problems (high anxiety, schizoid, paranoid, obsessive-compulsive behavior) or physical handicaps (growth retardation, orthopedic problems, speech and hearing problems). For youth who had suffered *severe* perinatal stress, the incidence of mental retardation was 10 times, the incidence of significant mental health problems was 5 times, and the incidence of significant physical handicaps was slightly more than twice that found in the total population of 18-year-olds.

Some residual effect of *moderate* perinatal stress was reflected in a greater incidence of mental retardation, significant mental health problems, and sociopathic (acting-out) behavior, especially among girls in adolescence. Incidence rates of significant physical health problems, and overall delinquency rates among those who had suffered from moderate perinatal stress, did not differ from the total cohort—but the incidence of significant mental health

Table 6 Problems at Ages 17–18 among Youth with Perinatal Stress

Problem	Total 1955 Cohort (%) (N=698)	Youth with Moderate Perinatal Stress (%) (N=69)	Youth with Severe Perinatal Stress (%) (N=14)
All problems	36.0	33.0	79.0
Mental retardation	3.0	6.0	29.0
Physical handicaps	6.0	6.0	14.5
Mental health problems*	3.0	9.0	14.5
Delinquency	15.0	17.0	21.5
Teenage pregnancies	6.0†	14.0†	0

* Schizoid, paranoid, obsessive-compulsive.
† Percentage of females.

problems was three times as high and that of mental retardation and illegitimate teenage pregnancies twice as high as that for all 18-year-olds on Kauai. Among the teenage pregnancies in this group were half of all the abortions. It should be pointed out, however, that in contrast to youth who had suffered from *severe* perinatal complications, the majority of those subjected to only *moderate* perinatal stress at birth were free of serious physical, learning, or behavior problems by age 18.

The following two cases illustrate these findings:

Case K. M.: This girl, with a rating of moderate perinatal stress, displayed head-banging as an infant and by age 2 was described as "anxious, awkward, bashful, dependent, dull, listless . . . inhibited, tense, and withdrawn." At age 10 her "air of depression" was noted on psychological evaluations with additional comment that it "could not even escape the casual observer." Mental health problems in adolescence were characterized by acting-out behavior—aggressive, antisocial behavior requiring frequent foster home placements and eventual commitment to the girls' school.

Case M. B.: This girl, with moderate perinatal stress, was always considered an extremely active infant, restless, not cuddly, and "like a stranger" to her mother. Diagnostic evaluation at age 10 resulted in recommendation for both LD placement and long-term mental health services. By then temper tantrums had increased and problems were noted in her distractibility and marked inability to concentrate, her negativism, her irritability, and her frequent lying and stealing. In adolescence she displayed severe behavior problems in school, requiring home tutoring. Eventually she withdrew, and at the time of our contact with her she indicated that school was of no importance to her, considered herself "undecided and confused," and expressed worry about her future.

In support of reports by Mednick and Schulsinger (1969) from Denmark and by Schachter (1950) from France on Caucasian samples, our findings provide both longitudinal and cross-cultural evidence that some significant mental health problems in late adolescence and young adulthood may be predictable in terms of a biological disposition in childhood and may be related to perinatal brain damage.

We found no statistically significant differences, by degree of perinatal stress, on the CPI or the Novicki Locus of Control Scale (I-E) at age 18. However, youth with severe perinatal stress who were not mentally retarded and could respond to the inventories had lower mean scores on the dominance, sociability, social presence, and self-acceptance scales of the CPI—all measures of self-assurance and interpersonal adequacy.

There were also no statistically significant differences, by degree of perinatal stress, on the verbal, quantitative, and total scales of the SCAT or the reading, mathematics, and writing scales of the STEP. It must be kept in mind, however, that the attrition rate for youth with moderate to severe stress was relatively high. About one-third of those who had suffered from severe perinatal stress were mentally retarded and unable to respond to these group tests because of their limited reading ability. Interestingly enough, those with perinatal stress scores of 3 who did take the tests had *higher* mean scores on both ability and achievement tests than youth with mild or moderate perinatal stress.

Our findings in a predominantly Oriental and Polynesian population are similar to those reported by Benaron et al. (1960) from a study of a predominantly black, low-SES sample. Their Chicago study also reported greater variability and a higher incidence of both below and above average intelligence among anoxic youth than among normal sib controls.

The Response of Community Agencies

In our report on the 10-year follow-up in the *Children of Kauai* (1971), we stressed the narrowing of the gap between the development of children with perinatal damage and their normal age peers from birth to middle childhood and ascribed this result to progress in medicine and the more general awareness of physical handicaps, resulting in an effective Crippled Children's Program. Our plea then was for greater attention to the needs of remedial education and mental health services, both for those with perinatal stress and those without who came from homes that could not provide for adequate educational stimulation and emotional security.

In the intervening years, youth who had suffered from greater perinatal stress had more frequent contacts with community agencies during adolescence than those with only mild or no perinatal complications. This was true for all agencies—with the exception of the Division of Mental Health. Differences by degree of perinatal stress were statistically significant for contacts with the Division of Vocational Rehabilitation and Rehabilitation Unlimited Kauai, with the Department of Health's Divisions of Mental Retardation and Public Health Nursing, and with the Department of Education's Office of Guidance and Special Services (see Table 7).

Among those with perinatal complications the mentally retarded had received the most painstaking attention. Positive actions in their behalf by the Health Department involved continuation of regular care begun in early childhood (12 percent), correction of persisting orthopedic conditions by surgery and braces (8 percent), and provision of medication and hearing aids (12 percent). The Department of Education's Special Services responded to their needs by placement of MRs in special classes (40 percent) and learning centers (8 percent) and by academic counseling (8 percent). Both agencies worked closely with Vocational Rehabilitation, which provided vocational counseling and guidance and placement in work-study programs (20 percent) or the Job Corps (4 percent) as well as prevocational evaluation and training and placement in the sheltered workshop of Rehabilitation Unlimited Kauai (4 percent). The record of intervention by a number of con-

Table 7 Percentage of 1955 Cohort with Agency Records by Age 18 by Degree of Perinatal Stress

Agency	None (%) (N=388)	Mild (%) (N=222)	Moderate (%) (N=69)	Severe (%) (N=14)	Chi Square*
Police	15.0	15.0	17.0	21.5	0.49
Family Court	6.0	8.0	7.0	14.0	2.32
Department of Health					
Public Health Nursing and Mental Retardation	7.0	3.0	9.0	14.0	7.60†
Mental Health	2.0	3.5	4.0	0.0	2.35
Department of Education					
Special Services	6.0	5.0	6.0	21.5	5.84†
Department of Social Services					
Vocational Rehabilitation	1.0	2.0	3.0	30.0	28.89**
Public Welfare	12.0	13.0	7.0	30.0	5.14
Total with agency contacts	33.2	32.4	30.4	50.0	2.08

* df=3.
† $p<.05$.
** $p<.01$.

cerned community agencies in behalf of the relatively small number of mentally retarded in this group reflects a spirit of excellent cooperation and, even rarer, a painstaking evaluation of individual progress. Case C. D., an educable mentally retarded young woman who suffered from severe perinatal stress, and Case A. B., a trainable mentally retarded young man with a record of severe perinatal complications, both from poor homes, are examples of differing degrees of success in intervention.

Case C. D.: This girl's birth history included severe preeclampsia, severe anemia, and near shock at delivery, necessitating oxygen and blood transfusion, in the mother, and cyanosis in the newborn. Her parents were poorly educated. The mother was rated "childlike, irresponsible, indifferent, erratic" and much family discord existed. The child was largely in the care of a senile and deaf grandmother. With a Stanford-Binet IQ of 64 and attendance in a special class for educable mentally retarded, she received only D's in reading, writing, and arithmetic. At age 10 she was placed in her first foster home and during the next five years was twice returned to her parents and twice placed in other foster homes. Running away from home, truancy problems in school, shoplifting, eventual withdrawal from school—this was the pattern. During this period she was involved in a work-study program under the auspices of the Vocational Rehabilitation Division. She had begun this program at age 14 (the earliest possible time under existing agency policies) as a result of recommendations made on the basis of our research panel's 10-year findings. Extensive notations exist of contacts with Public Welfare, Public Health Nursing, Vocational Rehabilitation, Family Court, Special Services, and counseling resources. Nevertheless, at age 17 she withdrew from school and is well along her path of repeating the cycle of irresponsibility, indifference, and erratic behavior.

Case A. B.: This boy was an illegitimate baby born by breech extraction who needed resuscitation. The child of a 16-year-old mother who was rated "unintelligent, childlike, irresponsible, suggestible," he showed severe retardation in mental development. At age 10 he had a Stanford-Binet IQ of 39 and a diagnosis of cretinism, hearing loss, and divergent strabismus. From age 7 on he participated in the training center program for severely retarded children. He was followed closely by the Department of Health's Child Development Clinics and the Department of Education's Special Services. At age 16 the Division of Vocational Rehabilitation started him in the workshop program of Rehabilitation Unlimited Kauai, where his adjustment was considered very satisfactory, and he continued to make good progress within the limitations of his ability. He currently participates in daily work there, meating coconuts, and is considered a contributing member of his sheltered workshop community.

The physical needs and, to some extent, the academic and vocational needs of youth who suffered from the long-term effects of birth complications were fairly adequately met. The mental health needs of such youth, however, have been less frequently recognized and even less adequately served. Fifteen percent of youth with severe perinatal complications had significant mental health problems in late adolescence, but none had any contact with community mental health agencies for diagnosis or treatment. Less than half (4 percent) the youth with moderate perinatal stress who had developed serious mental health problems in adolescence (schizoid behavior, obsessive-compulsive, paranoid, high anxiety) were seen by the Division of Mental Health. Only one received inpatient psychiatric treatment; the others were seen for diagnosis only.

There is no indication that pregnant teenagers in this group (including one whose father had committed incest and one who was pregnant at age 14) received any kind of positive counseling by community agencies—this includes the girls who underwent therapeutic abortions.

We noted that among the delinquents who had suffered from moderate or severe perinatal complications, there was a pattern of repeated, impulsive acting-out behavior (running away, truancy, shoplifting, traffic violations) characterized by a seeming inability to learn from experience and by extremely poor judgment. There were no records of attempts at counseling or behavior modification, except an occasional warning letter to parents by the Family Court or a reprimand by the police.

We need to keep in perspective that youth who develop serious mental health problems or sociopathic behavior are a minority among those subjected to moderate or severe complications at birth. Yet, by comparison with the much smaller proportion of mentally retarded, they have not received the attention they deserve. Since they seem doubly vulnerable because of an impaired biological disposition and a nonsupportive home environment, and since the likelihood of serious adult psychosis and sociopathy appears great (Kohlberg et al. 1972), we should have a greater awareness of their emotional and social needs at an earlier age.

CHAPTER 5
Learning Disabilities

Among the youth at risk from the 1955 cohort whom we followed through late adolescence were the 22 who, at age 10, had been considered in need of placement in a learning disability (LD) class. A panel consisting of a pediatrician, psychologist, and public health nurse had made the diagnosis of "probable MBD" and referral to an LD class at age 10 on the basis of the combined results of group and individual examinations (psychological and medical), grades, and behavior checklists filled out by teachers and parents independently (see *The Children of Kauai*, chap. 3). They used the following criteria:

1. Evidence of serious reading problems (i.e., reading more than one grade level below age expectancy) in spite of average (or above average) intelligence as demonstrated by performance on the Wechsler Intelligence Scale for Children (WISC)

2. WISC subtest scores characterized by a great deal of scatter with a significant (more than one standard deviation) discrepancy between verbal and performance IQ

3. Large number of errors, for age, on both the group and the individual Bender-Gestalt test (mean number of errors=4.5, Koppitz scoring)

4. Persistent hyperkinetic symptoms (extremely hyperactive, unable to concentrate, distractible) as judged by teacher, mother, and diagnostic evaluations

Detailed case studies of the 22 youngsters can be found in Appendix 3. Among these children, the proportion of boys (64 percent) was nearly twice that of the girls (36 percent). Among the major ethnic groups on the island, the Japanese were under-represented (18 percent among LDs; 33 percent in total cohort) and the Hawaiians and part-Hawaiians were overrepresented (36 percent among LDs; 22 percent in total cohort). A high propor-tion of LD cases came from homes rated low (50 percent) and very low (27 percent) in socioeconomic status; children from middle and upper SES homes were underrepresented (23 percent among LDs; 44 percent in total cohort).

Among the LD cases were four the panel considered to be in need of short-term mental health services (less than six months) and one who was considered to be in need of long-term services (more than six months). For the purpose of our analysis, all are treated as LD problems.

We carefully matched the LD cases with controls drawn ran-domly from the master list of 1955 births who were of the same sex and came from the same socioeconomic and ethnic back-ground, but who had no learning or behavior problems at age 10.

In this chapter we first examine differences between LD and control cases on selected variables at birth and ages 1, 2, and 10 and then focus on their status in late adolescence.

At Birth and Age 1

None of the LD cases in the cohort had suffered from *severe* peri-natal stress, but children who were later diagnosed as having learning disabilities had a higher proportion of *moderate* perina-tal complications (10 percent vs. zero), low birthweight (14 per-cent vs. 4.5 percent), congenital defects (9 percent vs. 4.5 percent), and chronic conditions judged by pediatricians as "possibly lead-ing to MBD" (13 percent vs. 5 percent) than the control cases of the same sex, SES, and ethnic group. Because of the small number of subjects involved in the comparisons, however, the differences between LDs and controls did not reach a statistically significant level.

At age 1, a higher proportion of mothers of infants who were later to become learning disabled rated their offspring as "*not* cuddly, *not* affectionate" (42 percent vs. 15 percent) and "*not* good-natured; fretful" (53 percent vs. 20 percent) than control mothers. These differences were significant at the $p < .05$ level. A lower proportion of future LDs than controls were seen by their mothers as "free of distressing habits" at age 1 (55 percent vs. 68 percent), but there were no significant differences in the proportion of infants in each group who were rated "very active" by their mothers (45 percent in each group). More mothers of infants who later were diagnosed as learning disabled were rated as "erratic" or "worrisome" (30 percent vs. none of the control mothers) by observers in the home; more control mothers were rated as "energetic" (25 percent vs. 10 percent), "patient" (25 percent vs. 10 percent), and "happy" (20 percent vs. 5 percent).

At Age 2

By the time the children had reached their second birthday, there were significant differences in infant behavior patterns and in parent-child relationships between the future learning disability and control cases. Ratings of both infant and maternal behavior were made by psychologists during the two-year examination without any knowledge of the birth records or one-year home observations. Children who later became learning disabled were characterized significantly more often by negative adjectives than control cases ($p < .02$)—adjectives such as "ambivalent," "awkward," "distractible," "fearful," "insecure," "restless," "slow," and "withdrawn." Controls were more often characterized as "agreeable," "alert," "calm," "quiet," and "responsive." Mothers of toddlers whose offspring were later to become learning disabled were described more often as "careless," "indifferent," or "overprotective"; control mothers were "kind," "temperate," "matter-of-fact," and "content." It is evident that a vicious cycle between a "nonrewarding" infant and an increasingly frustrated mother had begun in the first year of life and became aggravated in the second year.

There were also significant differences between future LD cases and controls on the Cattell Infant Intelligence Scale, which at age 2 is largely a measure of sensorimotor development (Cattell 1940) and the psychologists' rating of intellectual status. Thirty-seven percent of the toddlers who later became LD cases were judged below average by the psychologist on the basis of both test performance and behavior observations; another 26 percent were judged to be "questionable," in contrast to only 5 percent each of the control cases ($p < .01$). Mean Cattell IQs of future LD cases at age 2 were in the "slow learner" range (88); those of the control children were in the normal range (100). While differences between LDs and controls on the Cattell Infant Intelligence Scale were significant at the $p < .01$ level, mean differences between the two groups on the Vineland Social Maturity Scale (109 vs. 116) were less pronounced.

Independently of the psychological examination, pediatricians rated a higher proportion of future LD cases as below normal in physical development (24 percent vs. none in the control group). This difference was significant at the $p < .05$ level.

It appears that both psychological and pediatric screening in early childhood did identify a significant proportion of toddlers who later had serious learning problems in school (see *The Children of Kauai*, chap. 9).

The Home at Ages 2 and 10

At age 2, we evaluated family stability by using information from home interviews postpartum and at ages 1 and 2; these interviews gave evidence of family cohesiveness or upheaval and the type and duration of any instability. Of use was information on the legitimacy or illegitimacy of the child, presence or absence of the father, marital discord, alcoholism, emotional disturbance of parents, and long-term separation of child from mother without adequate substitute caretaker (see *The Children of Kauai*, chap. 4). Ratings ranged from very high or favorable (1) to very low or unfavorable (5). At age 2, there were no differences in the distribution of family stability ratings between future LD and control cases of the same sex, SES, and ethnic background.

At age 10, a clinical psychologist made ratings of the educational stimulation and emotional support provided by the home, ranging from very high (1) to very low (5), based on standardized interviews with the mothers conducted by two public health nurses and a social worker who were familiar with the community. The psychologist made the ratings without any knowledge of the birth history, the results of the 2-year and 10-year examinations, or previous ratings of family stability. (For a detailed description of the interview and assessment of the family environment, see *The Children of Kauai*, chap. 4).

We rated educational stimulation by considering the opportunities provided by the home for enlarging the child's vocabulary, the intellectual interests and activities in the home, the values the family placed on education, the work habits emphasized in the home, the availability of learning supplies, books, and periodicals, and the opportunities for exploring the larger environment (library use, special lessons, recreational activities). To rate emotional support we examined the information in the family interview on interpersonal relations between parents and child, on kind and amount of reinforcement used, on methods of discipline and ways of expressing approval, on the presence and absence of traumatic experiences, and on opportunities provided for satisfactory identification.

Though both LD and control cases were closely matched on ethnicity and socioeconomic status, a significantly higher proportion of LD children came from homes rated low and very low in educational stimulation (77 percent vs. 36 percent; $p < .025$) and rated low and very low in emotional support (68 percent vs. 28 percent; $p < .025$).

What has happened to the learning disability cases since puberty?

Contact with Community Agencies during Adolescence

In the span between ages 10 and 18, more than four-fifths of the youth diagnosed as LD cases at age 10 had some contact with community agencies. This rate exceeds that of any of the other "at risk" groups. It is nine times as high as that of controls matched by age, sex, SES, and ethnicity and nearly three times as high as that of the total cohort of 1955 births (see Table 8).

Differences between LDs and controls were highly significant for *total* agency contacts ($p < .001$), for contacts with the Department of Education's Office of Guidance and Special Services, and for contacts with the high school counselors ($p < .01$); and they showed a significant trend for contacts with the Department of Health's Division of Public Health Nursing, as well as for contacts with the police ($p < .10$).

One out of three LD cases (36 percent) was seen by the Department of Education's Special Services and the high school counselors because of poor academic record or poor attendance and truancy. One out of five (22.5 percent) was evaluated for possible placement in special classes. Only one was actually placed in a special learning center and work-study program, but one-third of all LDs received individual attention in regular classes, had curriculum adjustments, had speech therapy, or saw a professional counselor.

Only one out of five (18 percent) was seen for diagnosis by the Department of Health, Division of Public Health Nursing. It confirmed the presence of organic damage and learning disability but took no further action except for referrals to other agencies. Among them, the Division of Mental Health saw one out of every seven children with the LD syndrome (13.5 percent) for diagnostic purposes (learning problems, neurotic symptoms, problems with sexual identity), but only two received psychotherapy (9 percent) and only one received drug therapy (4.5 percent).

The most frequent contacts outside the school system for LD cases were with the judiciary system. Twenty-seven percent, nearly twice the rate for the total 1955 cohort, had contacts with the police, and half of these were repeated contacts that led to referral to the Family Court. Reasons included car accidents, malicious injury, larceny, burglary, running away from home, repeated truancy, curfew violations, and trespassing and unlawful hunting—generally a record of repetitive, impulsive, antisocial behavior.

Table 8   Differences in Agency Contacts During Adolescence Between LD Cases and Matched Controls

Agency	LD Cases (%) (N=22)	Controls (%) (N=22)	Chi Square*	p
Police	27.3	4.5	2.72	.10
Family Court	13.6	0	1.43	NS
Department of Health				
Public Health Nursing	22.7	0	3.61	.10
Mental Health	13.6	0	1.43	NS
Department of Education				
Special Services	36.4	4.5	5.03	.05
High school counselors	36.4	0	7.49	.05
Department of Social Services				
Vocational Rehabilitation	4.5	0	0	NS
Public Welfare (nonfinancial)	0	0	0	NS
Kauai hospitals†				
Teenage pregnancies	12.5	0	1.43	NS
Total with agency contacts	81.0	9	9.26	.001

* df=1.
† Females only.

Action taken by the judiciary system included placement on probation (9 percent), detention in the Hawaii Youth Correctional Facility (4.5 percent), placement in the Job Corps (4.5 percent), and in one case placement in the Hawaii State Mental Hospital.

There was no record of foster home placement by the Department of Social Services and Housing because of disturbed parent-child relationships, but rates of illegitimate teenage pregnancies for LD girls were twice as high (12.5 percent vs. 6 percent) as for females in the 1955 cohort.

Group Test Results at Age 18

Our results on the group tests taken in grade 12 confirm a picture of continued poor scholastic performance and serious under-achievement for youngsters diagnosed as LD cases in grade 5. There were significant differences between the LDs and control cases on *all* subtest and total scores of the SCAT (with the most pronounced difference on the verbal scale) and on *all* subtest scores of the STEP (with the most pronounced difference in reading and writing achievement). All differences were significant at the $p < .01$ level (see Table 9). Persistent visual-motor problems were noticed on individual Bender-Gestalt tests (mean number of errors=3; range 0 to 8). While there was some improvement on Bender-Gestalt scores on all but 2 of the 13 LDs on whom we were able to obtain individual scores at age 18, the results continued to indicate serious perceptual-motor problems.

On the threshold of adulthood, youths who had been diagnosed as LD cases at age 10 scored significantly lower than control cases on CPI measures of self-assurance and interpersonal adequacy, socialization and responsibility, and achievement potential and intellectual efficiency. At age 18, LD cases differed from control cases on the following CPI dimensions:

1. (Low) sociability ($p < .01$): identifies persons of outgoing, sociable, participative temperament

2. (Low) self-acceptance ($p < .05$): assesses factors such as a sense of personal worth, self-acceptance, and capacity for independent thinking and action

3. (Low) socialization ($p < .05$): indicates the degree of social maturity, integrity, and rectitude the person has attained

4. (Low) responsibility ($p < .01$): identifies persons of conscientious, responsible, and dependable disposition

5. (Low) tolerance ($p < .05$): identifies persons with permissive, accepting, and nonjudgmental social beliefs and attitudes

6. (Low) communality ($p < .05$): indicates the degree to which a person's responses correspond to the modal (common) pattern established by the inventory

7. (Low) achievement via independence ($p < .01$): identifies those factors of interest and motivation which facilitate achievement in a setting where autonomy and independence are positive behaviors

8. (Low) intellectual efficiency ($p < .05$): indicates the adequacy and effectiveness with which a person uses his or her intellectual resources

Because the dimensions of the CPI are intercorrelated, a discriminant function analysis was also run between the LD and control groups. The same subscales emerged as separating the two

Table 9 Means and Standard Deviations on SCAT, STEP, Locus of Control Scale, and CPI Dimensions Which Differentiate Significantly at Age 18 Between LD Cases and Matched Controls

Dimension	LD Cases at Age 10		Controls		t
	Mean	SD	Mean	SD	
SCAT	(N=12)		(N=13)		
Verbal	13.00	11.19	49.62	27.27	3.82*
Quantitative	18.33	18.77	52.00	35.01	2.86*
Total	12.82	13.87	50.23	29.40	3.01*
STEP	(N=11)		(N=16)		
Reading	13.46	12.38	41.31	28.33	2.95*
Mathematics	19.09	13.12	46.81	26.85	3.05*
Writing	9.64	8.05	50.06	28.96	4.34*
Locus of Control	17.8	4.8	12.1	3.7	3.34*
CPI scales	(N=14)		(N=18)		
Sociability	16.3	4.0	20.7	4.6	2.86*
Self-acceptance	15.5	4.1	18.9	3.9	2.37†
Responsibility	18.2	4.3	24.7	5.5	3.64*
Socialization	28.9	5.4	34.2	7.0	2.34†
Tolerance	11.1	5.0	15.7	5.1	2.55†
Communality	18.5	4.6	22.7	4.9	2.57†
Achievement via independence	10.3	2.9	15.5	4.1	4.03*
Intellectual efficiency	24.3	5.7	29.9	7.6	2.29†

*$p<.01$.
†$p<.05$.

groups to a significant extent. All variance was explained by one discriminant function, with the highest loadings on sociability, responsibility, and achievement via independence.

Noteworthy also was a highly significant difference between LD and control groups on the Novicki Locus of Control Scale ($p < .01$). The LD cases scored significantly more in the *external* direction (mean 18) than the controls (mean 12). The LD cases believed more strongly than controls that events were beyond their control and happened to them as a result of fate.

Interview Results at Age 18

At age 18, we were able to reach 90 percent of the cases who had been diagnosed as LD at age 10 and the same proportion of control cases. In Table 10 we present significant differences between the 20 LD cases and the 20 controls.

As can be seen from Table 10, both interview ratings (made by the psychologist at the end of the interview without any reference to other follow-up data, based on the total story and the youth's behavior) and specific answers to interview questions yielded a pretty dismal picture for the LDs that extended over

Table 10   Differences Between LD Youth and Matched Controls on Interview Dimensions at Age 18

Dimension	LD Cases (%) (N=20)	Controls (%) (N=20)	p*
Interview Ratings			
Participation in school activities (including extracurricular):			
(Very) limited	77	37	.05
Realism of educational plans beyond high school:			
Mixed—unrealistic	71	16	.001
Social life:			
(Very) good	30	70	.05
Degree of self-insight:			
(Very) little	53	7	.004
Goal and value differentiation:			
(Very) great	23	79	.001
Self-esteem:			
(Very) low	41	5	.006

Table 10   (Continued)

Dimension	LD Cases (%) (N=20)	Controls (%) (N=20)	p*
Interview Questions			
Interests and activities:			
Sports	80	100	.05
School-related organizations	10	45	.01
Educational plans:			
High school or less	45	15	.05
College or more	15	70	.004
Vocation considered:			
Plantation work	20	0	.05
Past and present employment:			
Plantation work	0	20	.03
Features of job deemed important:			
Interesting work	15	45	.05
Importance of doing well in school:			
High	20	50	.04
No close friends or confidants	53	15	.01
Parental goals for child:			
Father: academic	20	50	.05
Mother: academic	15	45	.04
Subject of family rules:			
Youth's whereabouts, hours of coming in	50	100	.003
Friends	0	20	.05
View of parental achievement demands:			
Father: college	20	50	.05
Mother: college	15	45	.05
View of parental understanding:			
Father: doesn't understand, at loss, unconcerned	42	15	.05
View of parental support:			
Mother: opposes, disagrees, uninterested	35	5	.05
Father: opposes, disagrees, uninterested	45	5	.002
Family closeness compared to friends:			
Family closer than friends	53	21	.04
Ways of changing self:			
Doesn't believe in change, sees no need	40	11	.05
Future goals and achievements:			
Happy, successful marriage	5	45	.004
Evaluation of help given:			
Of little help	57	19	.03

* Fisher's exact probability test.

many areas of their young adult life—for instance, their future plans:

> Maybe I'll try to go to college, any kind of college, as long as it is a place for learning.

> I might go to school . . . not sure . . . but just enough to get a good job. . . . I just want to get out of school now. . . . Well, it's all right . . . I don't know what I like about school, but there's nothing I don't like. . . . The way I think is that if you just pass, it's OK.

> No marriage for me. . . . I guess I'm not ready and don't know when I'll be ready.

As for their social life, in and out of school, and their view of parental support and understanding:

> We don't do much as a family, I'm afraid—we are only together if it's time for worries or when we eat. . . . My mother? She is nervous and overwrought, I guess that's about it. . . . When I was little they spanked me a lot when I did things wrong. . . . They scold me a lot, but don't spank anymore because they think I'm old enough to understand what's right and what's wrong. . . . My father? He's not that close to me. I don't know why but in the whole family I'm the only one he doesn't like—at least he acts that way. He always hassles and scolds me. [*Question*] My mother understands me pretty good. [*Question*] My father—I doubt it—he's still got his old ways.

> I spend more time by myself—my family and friends go out and I stay home more. . . . I don't feel I'm that close to my mother—nor my father. [*Question*] I like to be closer to myself since I'm all alone all the time anyway.

Regarding their (low) self-esteem and their (largely negative) evaluation of help given to them in the meantime, they had little to say. Questioned as to how people liked him, one LD youth said: "Not much. I'm slow." He described himself as "kinda shy." And when asked what he wanted most out of life, he shook his head: "I haven't thought of it. . . . Get a job or something." And later: "I'm satisfied with things as is—some people like you, some people don't. I just want to stay on this island." This youth was considered by the interviewer to be cooperative but very constricted. He saw no problems in life, had never gotten help from others, seemed to have settled into a passive acceptance of the status quo.

The LD cases were rated significantly lower than matched control cases on the realism of their educational plans ("mixed to unrealistic" for 71 percent); their participation in school-related activities ("very limited" for 77 percent); their present social life ("fair to poor" for 70 percent); the extent of their goal and value differentiation ("very low" for 77 percent); the degree of their self-insight ("very little" for 53 percent); and their self-esteem ("very low" for 41 percent).

In specific interview questions pertaining to education, a higher proportion of LD than control cases considered themselves as not doing as well as they should (35 percent vs. 10 percent), but a lower proportion assigned high importance to doing well in school (20 percent vs. 50 percent). A lower proportion of LD than control cases perceived academic accomplishments as parental goals and the same low proportion of LDs reported that their fathers and mothers wanted them to go to college. A much smaller proportion of LD than control cases chose college as their own goal and a much higher proportion were satisfied with high school education or less. With regard to future vocational goals, a lower proportion looked for "interesting work" in their vocational choice than job or career success.

While in school, most LDs appear to have been loners: A lower proportion had participated in both school and nonschool activities and a smaller proportion had participated in sports. Now, as young adults, more than half the LDs had no close friend or confidant and a much smaller proportion than control cases mentioned a "happy, successful marriage" as their future goal. Family involvement outweighed involvement with friends for a higher proportion of LD than control cases.

In spite of this "turning into" one's own family, a higher proportion of LDs than controls regarded both their mothers and fathers as nonsupportive, opposed, disagreeing, and uninterested in their plans—fathers more so than mothers. Fathers emerged as less understanding and less concerned and less influential over their offspring. A lower proportion of LD than control cases were very frank in discussing their fathers, and a lower proportion described their mothers in mainly positive terms.

Ironically, a higher proportion of LD cases than controls *without* problems did not believe in changing themselves and saw no need for improvement. The majority of the LD cases considered the assistance given to them by others (counselors, peers, professionals, teachers) as "of little help." The LDs' own evaluation of the effectiveness of the help given them may be fairly realistic. When we compare interview ratings of LD cases who received some form of positive intervention by community agencies (45 percent) with those who did not (55 percent), we find no significant differences.

Nine out of the 20 LD cases interviewed had received some help during adolescence: Six got help in the academic area (special class, learning center, speech therapy, home tutoring, work-study program) and two in the vocational area (placement in Job Corps or rehabilitation center); two received psychiatric counseling; one received drug therapy and another received treatment for a convulsive disorder. There were no sex or SES differences between treated or untreated LDs.

As can be seen in Table 11, the treated cases did have a higher proportion of youth rated high in achievement motivation, with a good social life and a greater extent of goal and value differentiation, than untreated LDs. Treated LD cases also had a lower proportion of youth with low self-esteem and great conflict feelings

Table 11   Differences Between Treated and Untreated Youth Diagnosed as LD Cases at Age 10 on Interview Ratings at Age 18

Dimension	Treated (%) (N=7)	Untreated (%) (N=11)	p*
Overall attitude toward school			
(very) favorable	57	73	.31
mixed reactions	29	27	
(very) unfavorable	14	0	
Achievement motivation			
(very) high	43	18	.22
content to get by	43	73	
(very) low	14	9	
Participation in school activities			
(very) extensive	0	0	.38
some	29	18	
(very) limited	71	81	
Realism of educational plans beyond high school			
(very) realistic	14	36	.27

Table 11 (Continued)

Dimension	Treated (%) (N=7)	Untreated (%) (N=11)	p*
mixed elements	86	64	
(very) unrealistic	0	0	
Job satisfaction			
(very) satisfied	50	75	.53
ambivalent	50	25	
(very) dissatisfied	0	0	
Social life			
(very) good	43	27	.31
fair	28.5	55	
(very) poor	28.5	18	
Feeling of security as part of family			
(very) strong	57	73	.31
fair	14	18	
(very) weak	29	9	
Identification with mother			
identifies (strongly)	86	73	.38
in conflict	14	18	
(very) rejecting	0	9	
Identification with father			
identifies (strongly)	57	73	.31
in conflict	0	9	
(very) rejecting	43	18	
Overall family adjustment			
(very) good	43	45.5	.37
fair	28.5	45.5	
(very) poor	28.5	9	
Degree of self-insight			
(very) high	14	27	.38
some	43	27	
little or none	43	45	
Extent of goal and value differentiation			
(very) great	43	27.5	.37
some	14	27.5	
little or none	43	45	
Intensity of conflict feeling			
(very) great	14	36	.27
some	72	28	
little or none	14	36	
Self-esteem			
(very) high	14	18	.47
fair	57	36	
(very) low	29	46	

* Fisher's exact probability test.

than untreated LDs. However, a majority of both the treated and the untreated LDs still were very limited in their participation in school activities, were not very realistic in their educational plans beyond high school, and had only a "fair to poor" social life and family life. Nearly half of all LDs, both the treated (43 percent) and the untreated (45 percent), had little or no self-insight, and less than one out of five in each group (14 percent vs. 18 percent) had a high self-esteem rating. This latter finding agrees with our estimates of overall rates of improvement, made by a comparison of 10-year status with the 18-year follow-up data. Only approximately one out of four (27 percent) were rated improved in status since age 10. Those LDs who did improve tended to have higher ratings of emotional support in their family than those who did not improve (see Chapter 10).

Discussion

Our findings, like those of the only other follow-up study of LDs with controls (Dykman et al. 1973), do not support the assumption that children with the LD syndrome will "grow out of their problems" during adolescence. For the overwhelming majority among the LDs diagnosed at age 10, problems persisted throughout adolescence and onto the threshold of young adulthood.

The record of agency contacts showed continuing problems in academic underachievement (confounded by absenteeism and truancy), a high incidence of repetitive, impulsive acting-out behavior that led to problems with the law and sexual misconduct during adolescence, and mental health problems that were less often recognized and attended to. On the threshold of adulthood, self-reports show a pervasive lack of self-assurance and interpersonal competency and a general inadequacy in using their intellectual resources. With a low self-esteem goes a feeling that one's actions are not under one's own control.

For most LDs diagnosed at age 10, family and friends are not seen as supportive or understanding—this impression seems to hold especially for LD sons in relationship to their fathers. Most LDs are loners, without close friends or confidants among peers, thrown back on the narrow circle of a family they view as nonsupportive.

There is a certain hopelessness about the efficacy of any outside help given them: Most judge attempts at positive intervention by counselors, peers, professionals, or teachers as being of "little help." Pervasive seems to be a lack of self-insight about one's own condition, coupled with no ability to see any need for change in oneself or belief in being able to effect change.

The few lucky ones who break out of this cycle—and there appear to be fewer in this group than among any other group of youth at risk (only about one out of every four)—seem to do so thanks to sustained emotional support that bolsters a fragile self-esteem. Earlier recognition of the LD problems, preferably at or even before school entry, is urgently needed if intervention by remedial education (Dykman et al. 1973) or drug therapy (Laufer 1971; Weiss et al. 1971) and psychiatric counseling (Mendelson et al. 1971) is to effect any significant improvement in status. Our data seem to indicate that the signposts are there and can be recognized by parents, pediatricians, and psychologists in infancy and early childhood:

Case R. J.: This girl was the second of seven children. Her perinatal stress score was zero, but the home received very low ratings in educational stimulation and emotional support during the early phase of our study. As an infant she was described as very active and cuddly, but she had the distressing habit of head-banging. The mother was noted to be "good-humored, reasonably relaxed, affectionate and considerate, taking things in stride." By age 2, the girl displayed hostile, restless, stubborn, and suspicious behavior and the mother had become indifferent and mildly ambivalent. The girl had a Cattell IQ of 74 and a Vineland SQ of 121 at this time; by age 10 her PMA IQ was 92. Individual psychological evaluation as well as group testing confirmed significant impairment in perceptual-motor functioning (WISC verbal IQ 82, performance IQ 62, full-scale IQ 70; error score of 8 on the Bender-Gestalt test), and recommendation was made for LD class placement. She was described at this time as distractible and stubborn, her feelings easily hurt, and her academic functioning poor.

At ages 11 and 12 the child was reported stealing at home and in school, was seen by a school counselor and the Mental

Health Service (the latter for drug and individual therapy), and participated in the Big Sister program. She was considered improved and treatment terminated.

By age 16 she was referred to the Family Court because she ran away from home and school; she was then placed under supervision of the court. Occasional acting-out behavior occurred, but she was considered to be responding well to counseling by her probation officer. School difficulties continued, however, and she cut classes, was suspended for gambling, and was failing her academic work. She became pregnant and had her baby just before the 18-year interview. The infant was cared for by her mother and she returned to school.

Interviewed in the last half of her senior year, after repeating a grade, her Bender-Gestalt error score was 8 and group test scores also confirmed perceptual-motor problems (SCAT verbal 29th percentile, performance 11th percentile). She was ambivalent about school: "I don't know how to explain. When we have so much work to do, that's the bad time, and good when the teacher doesn't assign so many assignments in one day." She did want to graduate, but had no further plans except a vague wish to work. She definitely had eliminated further schooling and thought that "maybe" she might get married.

Her own parents were divorced and she spoke very negatively of her father, but of her mother she said: "She's good—she treats us all right. I get along good with her, but not with my father." She felt "close enough" to her mother but "nothing" for her father. Anger and negative feelings accompanied these comments. She attributed much of her anger toward her father to his reaction to her pregnancy: "After he said I wasn't his daughter when I was pregnant . . . I got along OK before then." While she was growing up, her mother had stressed "no be like your father" and her father had stressed "nothing."

Her chief worry at this time related to whether her baby's father would come back and "the baby have her real father instead of a different guy." In spite of the agency records indicating professional help over the years, she insisted that only her "friends, my mother, and his mother" had helped her. Both she and her boyfriend had wanted her to have an abortion, but "my mother and his mother never liked me to have one and my friends never liked it, so I decided just to go through with it." She admitted to use of drugs over the years, including occasional hard drugs, but disavowed current use. She now considered premarital sex "junk," said that she and her boyfriend "knew, went to family class" but gambled that she would not become pregnant.

Earlier in the interview she had commented that her father's "gambling" had caused much family dissension in previous years. She added that she would tell her sisters to "enjoy life in a good way before they get married." She referred to herself as "just the usual me. [*Question*] I don't know—anyway. I get my moods—bad, good. [*Question*] I get uptight when I get all frustrated with things surrounding me." She was rated as "not improved."

Case D. V.: This male, born to a family of low socioeconomic status, was the youngest of 10 children and had a perinatal stress score of zero. He was considered fairly active as an infant and prone to temper tantrums and throwing himself on the floor. The mother was "good-humored, took things in stride, was rated affectionate, calm, patient." But she was also "careless and irresponsible." By age 2 the parent-child relationship was considered "matter-of-fact, indifferent, and distant," and the toddler was now described as "ambivalent, fearful, hesitant, persevering, and suspicious." His Cattell IQ was 107 and Vineland SQ 133.

At age 10 the home was rated as providing average educational stimulation and high emotional support. The boy was doing D work in school and was described by his teacher as unable to sit still, impulsive, and having unusual fears. Psychological evaluation yielded a WISC verbal IQ of 95, performance IQ of 85 and full-scale IQ of 89, with a Bender-Gestalt error score of 4 and significant subtest scatter on an earlier PMA test. He was recommended for LD class placement.

During his teen years he had no agency contacts and no special school services. His group test scores remained in the lowest 5 percent; his Bender-Gestalt score was still indicative of perceptual-motor problems. His curriculum had been adjusted to include primarily vocational courses. Interviewed in his senior year, he said that school was all right—"My senior year was the best, I only had to take a few courses"—and he was satisfied with his achievement. He planned to take a one-year trade course following graduation. For the previous two years he had worked as a busboy and very seriously reported that the main thing he hoped to achieve from life was "surfing."

He had never gotten help from anyone, but talked things over with friends from time to time (he had only a few friends) and did not feel he had any worries. He was only able to describe his parents in terms of their activities—"She likes to sew and stay home . . . he likes to go down to the beach." He indicated that he got along with them fairly well, but did not think himself similar to either parent nor have any desire to be like them. Their influence on him seemed primarily related to whether or not they let him go out: "They never did want me to go out too much, just stay home, but I always wanted to go out. . . . At least they let me go out pretty free now." His self-esteem was rated "fair"—"My personality is good enough, I guess. . . . I'm happy and satisfied with life"—and he expressed no feelings of conflict.

CHAPTER 6
Children in Need of Long-Term Mental Health Services

There were 25 youngsters in the 1955 cohort who, at age 10, were considered in need of long-term mental health services (six months or more). Their emotional problems had been identified through behavior checklists filled out independently by parents (usually the mother or stepmother) and teachers and confirmed by psycho-diagnostic tests and observations of clinical psychologists.

The overwhelming majority of the children in this group (80 percent) had acting-out problems: They were persistently aggressive; constantly quarreling and bullying; contrary and stubborn; destructive; lying; truant from home or school; or stealing. Other emotional problems mentioned were chronic nervous habits (tics; compulsive, persistent mannerisms; thumb-sucking, nail-biting, bed-wetting; stammering, stuttering, lisping) or persistent withdrawal (shyness, lack of confidence; feelings hurt easily; very unhappy, depressed most of the time; unusual fears and anxieties). Though some of the children also exhibited hyperkinetic symptoms, only one was judged to be in need of both placement in a learning disability class and long-term mental health services by the panel of pediatrician, psychologist, and public health nurse. The others were diagnosed as adjustment reactions of childhood, childhood neurosis, schizoid personality, or sociopathic personality. Their scores on intelligence tests were in the normal range (mean PMA IQ=94; SD=8.5). A description of the behavior mentioned by parents, teachers, and psychologists that led to the panel's diagnosis and recommendations is included in the case studies of the children in Appendix 3.

Among the children considered in need of long-term mental health (LMH) services, the proportion of boys (56 percent) was higher than the proportion of girls (44 percent). Of the major ethnic groups on the island, the Japanese and the Hawaiians and part-Hawaiians were underrepresented (16 percent of Japanese among LMH, 33 percent in total cohort; 16 percent of Hawaiians among LMH, 22 percent in total cohort). The Filipinos and especially ethnic mixtures, usually children of younger Japanese mothers and older Filipino fathers, were overrepresented (24 percent of Filipinos among LMH, 18 percent in total cohort; 36 percent of ethnic mixtures among LMH, 14 percent in total cohort). There were no children from the upper socioeconomic classes in this group, and the middle class was underrepresented as well (only 12 percent among LMH; 35 percent in total cohort). Children from lower socioeconomic classes, on the other hand, were considerably overrepresented (88 percent among LMH; 56 percent in cohort). As can be seen in Table 4, we succeeded in matching the long-term mental health cases with control cases of the same age and sex who came from the same ethnic background and the same socioeconomic status but had no behavior problems at age 10. There was, however, a significant difference in mean IQ between LMH and control cases on a group intelligence test (mean PMA IQ for controls=106; SD=9.2).

We will examine first some of the early differences between LMH and control cases at birth, in infancy, and in early childhood. Then we will focus on their status in late adolescence as revealed by both the public record (as judged by their contacts with community agencies during adolescence) and their private assessment of their own status (as judged by their responses to the 18-year interview).

At Birth and Age 1

There were no differences between children later diagnosed in need of long-term mental health services and control cases in the proportion of congenital defects (8 percent in each group). Among the LMH group there was, however, a higher proportion of low-birthweight babies, a higher proportion who had suffered from moderate to severe perinatal complications, and a significantly higher proportion of infants with "chronic conditions possibly leading to MBD" as judged by attending physicians. Twelve percent of the future LMH children weighed below 2,500 grams at birth in comparison with only 4 percent of the control cases. Twenty percent of the LMH cases suffered from moderate to severe perinatal stress as compared with 8 percent of the controls, and 44 percent were judged to have "chronic conditions possibly leading to MBD" in contrast to 16 percent of the control cases (chi square=3.63, df=1; $p < .10 > .05$).

At age 1, mothers of LMH infants rated a higher proportion of their offspring as "not cuddly, not affectionate" than control mothers (33 percent vs. 16 percent), but there were no significant differences between the two groups in maternal ratings of infants' activity level or the presence of distressing habits. Interviewers who observed the mothers at home characterized a higher proportion of mothers of future LMH children as "takes in stride" (60 percent vs. 42 percent of control mothers), "indifferent" (16 percent vs. 4 percent), "unintelligent" (16 percent vs. zero), "irresponsible" (12 percent vs. zero), and "discontented" (12 percent vs. 4 percent). A higher proportion of control mothers were described as "relaxed" (70 percent vs. 48 percent), "affectionate" (50 percent vs. 24 percent), "energetic" (42 percent vs. 28 percent), "happy" (33 percent vs. 12 percent), and "intelligent" (25 percent vs. 4 percent of LMH mothers).

Both at ages 1 and 2, mother-child relationships were described by a larger proportion of positive adjectives for control mothers (77 percent vs. 56 percent at age 1; 57 percent vs. 46 percent at age 2) and by a larger proportion of negative adjectives for mothers of future LMH children (42 percent vs. 22 percent at age 1; 41 percent vs. 31 percent at age 2).

At Age 2

By the time the children were seen for the two-year follow-up examinations, psychologists noted significant differences in parent-child relationships, infant behavior patterns, and the psychological status of the child between future LMH cases and controls. These observations, made without any knowledge of the birth records, mothers' ratings of their own infants at age 1, or ratings of the home interviewer, were based on observations before, during, and after the developmental testing with the Cattell Infant Intelligence Scale and the Vineland Social Maturity Scale.

Mothers of future LMH children were more often rated as

"matter-of-fact" (40 percent vs. 33 percent), "ambivalent" (16 percent vs. zero), and "hostile" (12 percent vs. zero) in their relationship to their children. Control mothers were more often characterized as "kind, temperate" (63 percent vs. 48 percent), "affectionate" (42 percent vs. 24 percent), and "content" (29 percent vs. 12 percent) but also more often as "restrictive" (17 percent vs. zero).

Toddlers who at age 10 were in need of long-term mental health services were more often characterized as "inhibited" (22 percent vs. 4 percent), "frustrated" (13 percent vs. zero), and "serious" (13 percent vs. zero) at age 2. Control children were more often described as "agreeable" (52 percent vs. 26 percent) and "responsive" (48 percent vs. 26 percent). Both the mothers' and the toddlers' behavior was more often described by positive adjectives for the control cases and by negative and "questionable" comments for the future LMH cases (chi square=2.71, df=1; $p < .10 > .05$).

There were no differences between the two groups in mean scores on the Vineland Social Maturity Scale nor in the psychologists' rating of intellectual status, but there was a significant difference in ratings of *psychological* status (chi square=3.97, df=1; $p < .05$). Some 27 percent of the future LMH children were noted to be below average (i.e., immature, emotionally unstable) at age 2 in comparison to only .05 percent of the control cases.

At age 2, there were no significant differences between future LMH cases and controls in the pediatrician's rating of physical status, but there was a higher proportion of both below normal ratings (17 percent vs. 9 percent) and superior ratings (13 percent vs. zero) among the future LMH cases than among controls. By age 10, the incidence of minor and moderate physical handicaps among children in need of long-term mental health services was three times as high as that of the controls (24 percent vs. 8 percent). Most common were psychosomatic complaints such as asthma and obesity.

The Home at Ages 2 and 10

Though control cases had been carefully matched with LMH cases on the basis of both ethnicity and socioeconomic status, the quality of the home environment differentiated them at both ages 2 and 10.

Already at age 2, a significantly higher proportion of future LMH cases (24 percent) came from homes rated low (12 percent) or very low (12 percent) in family stability. Though 88 percent of the control cases (the same proportion as among the LMH) came from the same poor and disadvantaged background, none of their families was rated low or very low in stability at age 2 (chi square=6.57, df=2; $p < .05$).

At age 10, more than four out of five LMH cases (84 percent), but only one out of every three control cases (33 percent), came from homes rated low in emotional support (chi square=13.15, df=2; $p < .01$). The same proportion of LMH cases (84 percent) came from homes rated low in educational stimulation in contrast to less than half (46 percent) of the controls (chi square=8.05, df=2; $p < .025$).

Case M. L.: This case presents a clear example of many of the distinguishing characteristics of the first 10 years of these youngsters' life span. Born with mild perinatal stress, the ninth of 11 children, he came from a home rated very low in socioeconomic status. Both educational stimulation and emotional support were rated very low. His mother was described during his infancy by home observers as "careless, indifferent, easygoing, unintelligent, childlike, irresponsible, erratic, . . . and impatient." When he was two years old, she was considered by a psychologist to be "easygoing, careless, matter-of-fact, and childlike." The infant was noted to keep to himself, with temperament and activity level "quiet," but he manifested head-banging. At age 2, with a Cattell IQ of 100 and a Vineland SQ of 113, he was described as "dependent, distractible, restless, and active." By 10 years, the mother labeled him a "troublemaker," constantly quarreling, stealing money from home and neighbors, unable to sit still. His fifth-grade teacher noted frequent stammering, uncontrolled emotions, bullying, lying, and stealing as well as destructiveness and academic difficulties. Psychological evaluation pointed to a bright youngster with poor emotional control as well as social difficulties. The immediate family history included mental retardation, child neglect, violent rages, and homicidal impulses as well as a suicide attempt by a sibling.

Contact with Community Agencies during Adolescence

What has happened to the children who needed long-term mental health services at age 10? Let us first take a look at their agency records during adolescence (see Table 12).

During the time span between age 10 and age 18, more than three-fourths (76 percent) of the youth considered in need of long-term mental health services at age 10 had contacts with community agencies, the majority as the result of persistent serious behavior problems. This rate of contact was more than six times as high as that for the controls matched by age, sex, SES, and ethnicity (12 percent). Differences between the LMH cases and controls were significant for total agency contacts ($p < .001$), contacts with the Division of Public Welfare ($p < .01$) and Division of Mental Health ($p < .02$). There was a significant trend in more frequent LMH contact with the Office of Guidance and Special Services ($p < .10$), with the police ($p < .10$), and, for the women among the LMH cases, with Kauai hospitals for teenage pregnancies and abortions ($p < .10$).

The highest percentage of contacts (one out of three) was with the police. The rate of contact of youth in need of long-term

Table 12   Differences in Agency Contacts During Adolescence Between LMH Youth and Matched Controls

Agency	LMH Cases (%) (N=25)	Controls (%) (N=25)	Chi Square*	p
Police	32.0	8.0	3.13	<.10
Family Court	16.0	0	2.45	NS
Department of Health				
Public Health Nursing	12.0	4.0	.27	NS
Mental Health	28.0	0	5.98	<.02
Department of Education				
Special Services	20.0	0	3.56	<.10
High school counselors	20.0	4.0	1.70	NS
Department of Social Services				
Public Welfare (nonfinancial)	32.0	0	7.29	<.01
Vocational Rehabilitation	4.0	0	0	NS
Kauai hospitals†				
Teenage pregnancies	20.0	0	3.56	<.10
Total with agency contacts	76.0	12.0	18.26	<.001

* df=1.
† Females only.

mental health services was four times that of controls matched by sex, ethnicity, and SES. They had more repeated contacts (16 percent) and more serious reasons for referral to the judiciary system than other groups at risk. The most frequent reasons were larceny, burglary, assault and battery, drug abuse, running away from home, and sexual misconduct. One out of six youngsters (16 percent) in need of long-term mental health services at age 10 were referred to the Family Court during adolescence. They were placed in detention, in the Job Corps, or in custody of the Division of Public Welfare.

Only one out of every four of those needing long-term mental health services at age 10 were seen by the Division of Mental Health during adolescence (28 percent), and less than one out of ten (8 percent) ever received any therapy, either individual psychotherapy (8 percent) or drug therapy (4 percent). The remainder were seen for diagnostic workups only and were referred to other local agencies. Diagnoses made by the Mental Health Division included neurotic problems, psychosomatic problems, problems with sexual identity, and borderline psychoses (undifferentiated schizophrenia), in addition to adjustment reactions and transient situational behavior disorders. None of the control cases was considered to need mental health services.

The Division of Public Welfare saw nearly one out of three of the youth needing long-term mental health services, either because of behavior problems or disturbed parent-child relationships or because they had become a custody case. One out of every four (24 percent) was eventually placed in a foster home. None of the control cases needed nonfinancial assistance by Public Welfare.

The schools, both through the Office of Guidance and Special Services and the counselors in the three high schools, saw only one out of every five (20 percent) of the youth in need of long-term mental health services, but they did provide services for everyone they saw. Reasons for referrals were either truancy, coupled with a poor academic record (inspite of normal intelligence), or discipline problems (including drinking, drug abuse, and gambling on school premises during school hours). Only one control case had a truancy problem.

The Division of Public Health Nursing had contacts with one out of every eight of the youth in need of long-term mental health services, mostly because of orthopedic handicaps and needs for surgery which were met by the actions taken through the Department of Health. Their rate of contacts with Public Health Nursing was three times as high as that for the controls (12 percent vs. 4 percent).

Among the girls in this group, one out of five (20 percent) had had an illegitimate pregnancy during adolescence, in contrast to none of the girls in the control group. This rate of teenage pregnancies among girls formerly diagnosed in need of long-term mental health services was nearly three times as high as that for all women in the 1955 cohort. This was also the group at risk with the highest rate of abortions (10 percent, or half of all the pregnancies in this group). Several of these youngsters were involved with multiple agencies. The following case is an example:

> **Case A. C.:** At age 11½ she was known to the police and referred to Family Court, Mental Health, and the Crippled Children's Branch of the Health Department. By age 12 the Department of Social Services and Housing and the Family Court were involved in planning and service. Between ages 12 and 15 there were annual evaluations by the Division of Public Welfare with referral to the Department of Health for intermittent health problems. From ages 15 to 17, the Department of Social Services and Housing, Mental Health, private medical facilities, and the Crippled Children's Branch were involved in extensive evaluations and treatment. Withdrawal from school occurred at 16½ years with police contacts regarding burglary and drug abuse following. At age 17 the Division of Public Welfare's custody was revoked, and at the time of the interview she was found to be undecided in her future plans but insistent that they include freedom from supervision and a freedom to develop her own ideas.

Group Test Results at Age 18

There was a high attrition rate among youth in need of long-term mental health services who took the group tests of ability, achievement, and interpersonal competency in grade 12. Although we arranged for repeat test sessions and also distributed the personality test after the interview to those who had not taken it, only 52 percent (13 out of 25) of the LMH cases took the SCAT and the STEP and only 14 (56 percent) took the CPI and the Locus of Control Scale. At each group test session, there was a higher rate of absenteeism among the youth in need of long-term mental health services than among other groups of youth at risk. This absenteeism is reflected also in the truancy reports of the principals and counselors in the three high schools. Hence the results of the group tests need to be taken with a grain of caution.

On the SCAT, the LMH youth who did take the test scored significantly lower than controls on the verbal and the total scale ($p < .01$ and $p < .05$ respectively). While mean scores of the controls were about average on all SCAT scales, LMH cases averaged around the 20th percentile on the verbal and total scale and slightly higher (26th percentile) on the quantitative scale. A similar trend was found on the STEP in grade 12: Controls had means around the 50th percentile on the reading and writing scale; LMH cases averaged around the 20th percentile and scored higher (around the 36th percentile) in mathematics. Differences between the controls and LMH cases were statistically significant on the reading scale ($p < .01$) and writing scale ($p < .01$) of the STEP, but not on the mathematics scale.

Only slightly more than half (56 percent) of the LMH youth responded to the CPI and the Locus of Control Scale. Those who did respond had similar mean scores as the controls on both tests. This was the only group of youth at risk which was not differentiated by t tests or discriminant function analysis on any of the CPI subscales from the controls. We are inclined to ascribe the lack of significant differences to a high absentee rate among the serious behavior problems and to defensiveness and evasiveness among those who did cooperate. There was also a higher proportion of refusals and repeated broken appointments among the LMH cases than any other group of youth at risk when we contacted them for a personal interview at age 18.

Interview Results at Age 18

We present here the findings from the interviews with 20 LMH and 20 control cases we were able to interview. This presents 80 percent of the original sample (an additional case, diagnosed as having both a learning disability and serious behavior problems, was included in the statistical analysis of the learning disability cases).

As can be seen from Table 13, there were a number of significant differences at age 18 between the youth considered in need of long-term mental health services at age 10 and matched control cases. Most dealt with the quality of their family and peer relationships.

A significantly lower proportion of LMH youth than controls was still living with both natural parents (74 percent vs. 95 percent), and a much smaller percentage of the LMH youth chose either parent as a model for what they wanted to be (29 percent vs. 56 percent). Although a higher proportion of LMH youth than controls thought that their mother had influenced them much (44 percent vs. 20 percent), a significantly lower proportion viewed themselves as similar to their mothers in personality (18 percent vs. 62 percent). A significantly higher proportion of the LMH youth, however, saw their father in a positive way (60 percent vs. 25 percent) and stressed that their father had "moral" goals for them (44 percent vs. 20 percent)—i.e., to "be and do good."

Table 13   Differences Between LMH Youth and Matched Controls on Interview Dimensions at Age 18

Dimension	LMH Youth (%) (N=20)	Controls (%) (N=20)	p*
Participation in school activities (including extracurricular):			
Very limited	50	17	.03
Features of job deemed important:			
Interesting work	26	60	.04
Friends:			
Many	50	20	.05
Makeup of nuclear family:			
Living with both natural parents	74	95	.04
Tone of description of father:			
Positive	60	25	.05
View of similarity to parents:			
Similar to mother	18	62	.04
View of parental achievement demands:			
Father: college	25	55	.05
Weak points:			
"Low self-esteem"	33	—	.01
Psychotherapy:			
Considered it, went regularly	40	11	.05
Evaluation of help given:			
Helped a lot	53	40	NS
Helped a little	33	47	NS

* Fisher's exact probability test

Typical of the comments were these from a female LMH case:

> My mother? She's the sweetest thing in the world. . . . It's funny how she can even cope with me. . . . She's influenced me a lot. . . . She's a good housewife and mother. Without her I won't be interested in nursing. [*Father*?] Mother's the main influence. . . . He can sing and play instruments. He taught me to sing, dance and fight. . . . She wants me to be something that will make me happy. . . . He wants me to be a secretary, to behave.

And a male control responded in this way:

> My mother? She's very emotional, concerned about everything, and a little hot-tempered, but very loving and considerate. My father is about the same, but a little prouder. I like him. I think everyone should admire his father, someone to look for in authority. . . . I'm not like either of them, I'm different, I'm myself. . . . They've influenced me just about right and wrong—they're sort of religious and we were brought up within our religion. . . . They have influenced me about matters of respect and honor, but not about future endeavors . . . that I've learned in school. . . . They never told me what to do or what to be, and I thank them for it.

Fathers' achievement demands were perceived as lower by the LMH youth than by the control youth. Only 25 percent of the LMH youth stated that their fathers wanted them to go to college, in contrast to more than half (55 percent) of the controls. Their own ambitions, both educationally and vocationally, were more limited. Only half the proportion of LMH compared to control cases planned to go to college (35 percent vs. 70 percent). A significantly lower proportion of LMH youth than controls considered "interesting work" an important feature of the job they would choose (26 percent vs. 60 percent), and only a third had definite vocational plans (33 percent). Those who did preferred "skilled trade" over other options (40 percent of LMH vs. 10 percent of controls). Though about half the LMH youth interviewed claimed they had "many friends" (50 percent vs. 20 percent of the controls), a much smaller proportion among the LMH than the controls had a steady boyfriend or girlfriend (5 percent vs. 25 percent) and a smaller proportion was interested in social activities that involved both the same and the opposite sex (61 percent vs. 84 percent). Peer friends, however, were considered a source of help by a considerably higher proportion of LMH youth than SMH youth (67 percent of LMH vs. 36 percent of SMH).

Regarding the list of their weak points, "bad temper" differentiated the LMH cases from the controls, but not in the expected direction (6 percent vs. 33 percent). One-third of the LMH cases were rated as low in "self-esteem" (33 percent) in comparison with none of the controls. As some LMH subjects remarked:

> Well, I'm just a person in the world—one person trying to find his goal in the near future.

> I'm a follower. I think I'm sensitive, I'd like to be smarter, I think I'm stupid. I'd like to be skinnier.

> I don't know—I'd describe myself by my age—I don't know. [*Question*] I'm lost, this is just like hell itself.

> I don't know—nothing—don't know what I am . . . think I'm not happy. [*Question*] Half-half, but I don't know if I could change.

> I don't know. . . . I could say I'm unpredictable. . . . I wish I had studied harder. . . . I fool around too much.

And in contrast, controls had this to say:

> First of all, I respect other persons. I'm a person to look up to. . . . I have a sense of humor, personality, physically OK. . . . I like to play sports, lots of kids look up to me. Come around me. Maybe—just *maybe*—I'm a person with good looks [*he was a handsome boy*].

> I'm not too dumb. I know enough to get around, take care of myself . . . have average intelligence. If I was putting in a want ad, I'd mention other things. . . . I'm a firm believer in God. . . . I follow the law. I'm living so I won't be put in jail anyway!

> I'm friendly, some people say, and I like to do lots of things and I'm interested in becoming a nurse to help others.

In contrast with the learning disability cases, a higher proportion of youth for whom long-term mental health services were recommended by professionals at age 10 saw this need in themselves during adolescence. Eight of the interviewed cases (40 percent of interviewees, 33 percent of total LMH sample) stated that they had considered psychotherapy and went occasionally or regularly for outside help, a number that agrees with our records of positive intervention by agencies in the community. This proportion differs significantly from the control cases (none of whom had any psychotherapy) and from the short-term mental health cases (only 15 percent of whom thought they needed psychotherapy).

There were no significant differences between LMH and control cases in their evaluation of the outcome of help given to them, but about half (53 percent) of the LMH cases said "it helped a lot," a proportion that corresponds closely to the improvement rate among the treated LMH cases (1:2) and is more encouraging than the predominantly negative evaluation of the outcome of help given to the learning disability cases.

When we compare interview ratings of the few LMH cases (33 percent) who received some form of positive intervention (counseling, individual psychotherapy, drug therapy, foster home placement, corrective surgery) with those who did not (66 percent), we find no statistically significant differences between the two groups but some trends that are encouraging (see Table 14). A higher proportion of treated than untreated LMH cases had a (very) good social life (75 percent vs. 50 percent) by age 18. A higher proportion had a (very) strong feeling of security as part of their family (75 percent vs. 50 percent). All treated cases identified strongly with their mothers (100 percent vs. 64 percent) and most with their fathers (75 percent vs. 46 percent): The majority of treated LMH cases had a (very) good family adjustment (75 percent vs. 43 percent) by age 18. The proportion of those with a (very) high degree of self-insight was considerably higher among the (few) treated than among the untreated LMH (50 percent vs. 21 percent).

Among the treated LMH cases there was also a higher proportion with (very) high self-esteem (50 percent) than among the untreated (14 percent) and a lower proportion with intense conflict feelings (25 percent vs. 36 percent). Most significantly, the extent of present goal and value differentiation, at the threshold of adulthood, is higher ($p < .08$, Fisher's exact probability test) among the treated than among the untreated LMH (75 percent vs. 21 percent).

Estimates of overall rates of improvement, made by a comparison of 10-year status with all 18-year follow-up data, including agency records, are higher for the treated LMH cases (1:2) than for the untreated (1:4). Overall rates for improvement for LMH youth were, however, still discouragingly low: Only one out of

Table 14   Differences Between Treated and Untreated LMH
Youth on Interview Ratings at Age 18

Dimension	Treated (%) (N=4)	Untreated (%) (N=14)	p*
Overall attitude toward school			
(very) favorable	25	64	.18
mixed reactions	50	22	
(very) unfavorable	25	14	
Achievement motivation			
(very) high	25	36	.43
content to get by	50	57	
(very) low	25	7	
Participation in school activities			
(very) extensive	25	14	.31
some	0	36	
(very) limited	75	50	
Realism of educational plans beyond high school			
(very) realistic	50	64	.38
mixed elements	50	29	
(very) unrealistic	0	7	
Job satisfaction			
(very) satisfied	50	80	.48
ambivalent	0	20	
(very) dissatisfied	50	0	
Social life			
(very) good	75	50	.31
fair	0	43	
(very) poor	25	7	
Feeling of security as part of family			
(very) strong	75	50	.31
fair	0	14	
(very) weak	25	36	
Identification with mother			
identifies (strongly)	100	64	.23
in conflict	0	36	
(very) rejecting	0	0	
Identification with father			
identifies (strongly)	75	46	.28
in conflict	0	23	
(very) rejecting	25	31	
Overall family adjustment			
(very) good	75	43	.25
fair	0	14	
(very) poor	25	43	
Degree of self-insight			
(very) high	50	21	.25
some	25	43	
little or none	25	36	

Table 14 (Continued)

Dimension	Treated (%) (N=4)	Untreated (%) (N=14)	p*
Extent of goal and value differentiation			
(very) great	75	21	.08
some	0	43	
little or none	25	36	
Intensity of conflict feelings			
(very) great	25	36	.43
some	50	28	
little or none	25	36	
Self-esteem			
(very) high	50	14	.18
fair	25	64	
(very) low	25	22	

* Fisher's exact probability test.

three (8 out of 24; 4 of the 8 treated and 4 of the 16 untreated) had improved their status by the end of adolescence (see Chapter 10).

Discussion

Our follow-up data regarding youth who had been considered in need of long-term mental health services at age 10, gathered at the threshold of adulthood, can lend themselves to either an optimistic or a pessimistic interpretation, like the proverbial glass half full (or half empty) of water. On the positive side, and this is the lesson we learned from our controls and from those among the LMH youth who improved, it appears that belonging to a "nonwhite culture of poverty" does not inevitably lead to trouble in one's community. We say this with a great deal of respect for the resiliency of the human spirit against all odds.

To illustrate: The overwhelming majority of our youth at risk (more than four-fifths of those in need of long-term mental health services at age 10) came from poor homes, yet the percentage of recorded problems with the system (police and courts, schools and public welfare agencies) for the controls, who came from the same socioeconomic background and ethnic groups, was minimal. Among the controls only 8 percent had committed any delinquent acts, only 4 percent presented achievement or discipline problems in school, and none had needed referral to the Division of Mental

Health for behavior problems during the turbulent period of adolescence. None of the controls revealed any pathological symptoms on the California Psychological Inventory and only two saw any need for psychotherapy in the clinical interview at age 18.

Our findings with the predominantly Oriental and Polynesian youth of Kauai in the 1970s support the conclusions drawn by Robins on the basis of her follow-up of lower-class whites (1966) and blacks (1970) who attended urban St. Louis elementary schools in the 1920s and 1930s: "Low social status in childhood does *not* predict severe and pervasive antisocial behavior in adulthood. Families can live in slums and be on relief rolls *without* their children responding to the frustrations of poverty or the examples of delinquency in their neighborhood with sociopathic behavior" (Robins 1966:198).

The second encouraging finding, though it is unfortunately based on the minority (33 percent) of youth who obtained the help they needed, is that some form of positive intervention by community agencies or volunteers, whether in the form of counseling, tutoring, psychotherapy, drug therapy, or an affiliation by a concerned peer, can apparently contribute to improvement.

Let us now look at the outcome of those *not* treated: Only one out of four shows any apparent improvement since age 10. Three out of four still have serious problems at age 18. This, then, brings us to the more pessimistic aspect of our findings: The overwhelming majority (two out of three) of those who in early elementary school were considered in need of long-term mental health services continued to have serious behavior and learning problems in adolescence and up to the threshold of adulthood. Kauai's youth of many races who had need of long-term mental health services at age 10 showed a variety of antisocial disorders during adolescence that are very similar to the deviant children grown up in Robins' study of urban whites (1966) who were referrals to child guidance clinics.

The distressing aspect of *our* findings is the continuity of serious behavior problems among those who, in middle childhood, had for the most part had acting-out problems. Their story, as it unfolds in adolescence and young adulthood, is reminiscent of the defeated lives of the sociopathic adults who were followed by

Robins (1966) in middle age. Psychosomatic and psychotic symptoms (especially schizoid behavior), sexual misconduct or problems with sexual identity, assault and battery, theft and burglary, drinking and drug abuse, and continued poor academic performance coupled with absenteeism and truancy left these youth few options for a satisfactory education or vocation or for social and personal development in later years. Since generally they did not view parents as satisfactory models for identification, the influence of peers prevailed, for better or worse. The majority recognized a need for therapy, but turned to their peers for the help they did not obtain or seek from professionals or their families.

Looking back into their early lives, it becomes apparent that a sizable proportion of these youths were doubly vulnerable—products of an impaired biological disposition recognizable at birth and products of frustrated parental responses to a nonrewarding infant and toddler in a family setting that was already unstable in early childhood.

Unfortunately, the proportion of children among those needing long-term mental health services in elementary school who received some attention by the Division of Mental Health is low (28 percent). It is identical with the small proportion among child guidance clinic referrals in the 1920s and 1930s who received any treatment (Robins 1966:210). The total proportion for whom there was any kind of positive intervention by community agencies—one out of three—is the same percentage that emerged from Levitt's review (1971) of some 47 reports of the outcome of psychotherapy spanning a 35-year period from the 1920s through the late 1960s. Both reports cover time spans before any widespread federal, state, and local concern (and public expenditure) for early screening and the community mental health approach. If this present concern, as evidenced by recent federal and state legislation (among them the 1970 Developmental Disabilities Act), is to be translated into effective action, children having the serious mental health problems described in this chapter should be among our top priorities for early detection and positive intervention. They need our public resources and personal commitment desperately. Some improvement, brought about by diagnosis and intervention in middle childhood, is reflected in the lessened intensity of conflict, greater insight, higher self-esteem, and greater goal and value differentiation among the few in our sample who have obtained help through educational, mental health, and social agencies and concerned volunteers.

Our data suggest that this positive intervention needs to be broadened to include more of the childhood acting-out problems and that the recognition of potential significant mental health problems might well begin with a look at the biological and temperamental disposition of the child at birth and the quality of parent-child relationships in infancy and early childhood—before the problem has gained an irreversible momentum:

> **Case Z. Y.:** This boy, the oldest of two children (perinatal stress score=1), was described in infancy as not liking affection, a baby who was fairly active and did considerable head-banging. The mother, considered "intelligent, energetic, self-controlled, and self-confident" in his infancy, was described as "irritated" by age 2 and the toddler as "frustrated, sensitive, serious, and tense." His Cattell IQ was 91 and his Vineland SQ was 126.
>
> By age 10 his mother noted him to be fearful and anxious and "depressed most of the time." He lied frequently and was a truant from school. His fifth-grade teacher considered him extremely irritable, bullying, and constantly quarreling, and his academic achievement was unsatisfactory. Individual psychological testing yielded a WISC full-scale IQ of 112, a verbal IQ of 104, and a performance IQ of 118, though results of group tests were lower (PMA IQ=99). His frustration tolerance was limited, his behavior impulsive and hostile with only limited ego control. The psychologist noted at that time: "I consider him to be a more than moderately disturbed child whose aggressive and hostile-defensive behavior is an expression of unmet needs for affection and understanding at home."
>
> Recommendations were made for psychiatric and social work services as well as temporary foster home placement in the event of further personality breakdown. The home situation had apparently deteriorated over the years with frequent family fights, alcoholism, attempted suicide by the mother, and eventual divorce of the parents. Following the death of his father, who had been awarded custody of the youngster,

he was placed in a foster home. He continued to manifest signs of depression and acting-out behavior. Police contacts for shoplifting, theft, complaints of assault, and drinking filled his adolescent record. Intervention efforts consisted in foster home placement and occasional contacts with the school counselor.

At age 18 the boy indicated that "there are people with problems and people without, and I don't have any. I like the life I'm leading now. . . . I got help the time I got caught drinking beer but I don't think I ever had problems. I learned a lot from my friends. . . . I didn't think I needed any other help. . . . I don't want to say any more." (The interviewer noted that he was extremely restless and uncomfortable.) At the time of the interview, three weeks before high school graduation, he did not know what he wanted to do after finishing high school but thought he might go to the local community college. He could not describe any strong or weak points about himself, had no long-term goals, and expressed little optimism about the future. He was rated as "not improved."

Case W. X.: This boy (perinatal stress score=0) was the youngest of five children. He was born into a family rated very low in socioeconomic status, educational stimulation, and emotional support. In infancy he was considered fairly active and clinging to his mother, who was described as "easygoing, indifferent, irresponsible, negativistic, and discontented." By age 2 the toddler was considered "bashful, dull, fearful, dependent, listless, passive, and inhibited," while the mother's relationship with her son impressed observers as "indifferent, distant, hostile, careless, and childlike."

Although it was apparently not noted then, information obtained later, at the time of the 10-year follow-up, revealed that the mother had been diagnosed as schizophrenic at age 19 and had been mentally ill since that time. She had been in and out of hospitals and was always particularly depressed during and after her pregnancies; her care of the children had been haphazard. The father had limited understanding of her condition and had difficulty meeting the needs of the children, all of whom were considered products of cultural impoverishment and inadequate parenting. The boy had a Stanford-Binet IQ of 106, but as a 10-year-old he was performing unsatisfactorily in his academic work. His fifth-grade teacher described him as very slow of speech, distractible, and having a very short attention span—a depressed, unsmiling boy who lacked self-confidence and did not participate well in group activities.

Until age 12 he was followed intermittently by the Department of Social Services and Housing, but the case was closed at that time with his condition reported as "stabilized." His mother's death shortly thereafter left a household of three boys and the father. When interviewed in adolescence he indicated that most of his time was spent with friends in his church group and that he had been active with the group since grade 7. The family was apparently very much involved with one of the fundamentalist religions, and the youth derived his major support and values from the group. His own plans for the future involved ministerial work with the group, with whatever part-time work he could get as a means of self-support. He considered the church to be the major influence in his life.

Speaking of his parents, he said he did not know how to describe his father but after a long pause said: "He's all right—he was kind of carefree, never really cared for us, and my mother worried a lot." He indicated that he had respect for his mother but never really knew her. Referring to her mental illness, he said: "She was mentally disturbed, I think." He wondered about her influence on him: "It's almost natural for you to inherit things from your parents."

He felt that he worried about himself as a person but solved most of his problems by himself. Although he had not gotten into any trouble during his teen years, he indicated that school was a waste of time and he did just enough to pass. He described himself as "different from most people" and his outlook for the future was relatively pessimistic. He felt things "will become pretty bad in the world, but not to the extent of total destruction." He saw an eventual "new order" and indicated his goal would be "to get into the new order"—"Problems will be solved, but not by man, that way

I don't have to worry about things.'' Certainly this young-ster's conflict was lessened through intervention of concerned volunteers and the support of friends in his church. One can only speculate what the outcome might have been with greater attention to the early parent-child relationships.

CHAPTER 7
Children in Need of Short-Term Mental Health Services

Among the 1955 cohort there were 60 children (about 10 percent) who at age 10 were considered in need of short-term mental health (SMH) services by the panel of pediatrician, psychologist, and public health nurse who reviewed the results of our screening and diagnostic tests. All these children were diagnosed as "adjustment reactions of childhood," and it was felt that some mental health service (of less than six months' duration) would be beneficial to them.

Appendix 3 summarizes the behavior descriptions by parents, teachers, and psychologists that led to the diagnoses and recommendations. The overwhelming majority in this group were shy, anxious children who lacked self-confidence and had developed chronic nervous habits to deal with their insecurities. There was a much smaller proportion (20 percent) of acting-out problems in this group than among those considered in need of long-term mental health services (80 percent). Four of the 60 were considered both to have learning disabilities and to be in need of short-term mental health services (they were included in our analysis of the learning disability cases in Chapter 5). There was an equal number of boys (30) and girls (30) among those in need of short-term mental health services. Of the major ethnic groups on the island, the Japanese were underrepresented (14 percent among the SMH; 33 percent among the 1955 cohort) and the Portuguese were overrepresented (12 percent among the SMH; 6 percent among the 1955 cohort).

There were fewer children from the middle class in this group (24 percent among SMH; 35 percent in the 1955 cohort) and children from poorer homes were overrepresented (71 percent among SMH; 54 percent in the 1955 cohort), but not quite as disproportionately as among the children with learning disabilities and those in need of long-term mental health services. We matched the short-term mental health problems with control children of the same sex, socioeconomic status, and ethnic group from the 1955 cohort who had no behavior problems at age 10. We contrasted these two groups in the analysis of our data from birth, infancy, and childhood and the agency records and group test results in adolescence. Limitations of time did not allow us, however, to interview the control cases at age 18; hence the interview results for the short-term mental health cases will be contrasted with those from youth with severe behavior problems in need of long-term mental health services at age 10. Let us first take a look at the early data and then focus on the status of the short-term mental health problems in adolescence and young adulthood.

At Birth and Age 1

In contrast to the learning disability cases and long-term mental health cases, there were no significant differences between infants later diagnosed in need of short-term mental health services and controls in incidence of perinatal complications, congenital defects, or low birthweight. A slightly higher proportion of SMH infants were rated "not cuddly or affectionate" by their mothers at age 1 (20 percent vs. 7 percent of controls). By age 2, a higher proportion of later SMH children was characterized as "dependent" (30 percent vs. 14 percent), "hesitant" (21 percent vs. 12 percent), and "inhibited" (22 percent vs. 2 percent). Controls were more often described as "agreeable" (39 percent vs. 26 percent) and "alert" (24 percent vs. 12 percent) by the psychologists who observed the children before, during, and after the developmental examinations.

Mothers of future SMH children were more often characterized as "childlike" (15 percent vs. 7 percent) and "warmhearted" (51 percent vs. 32 percent) by observers who saw them in the home; control mothers were more often described as "resource-ful" (22 percent vs. 10 percent).

At age 2, psychologists characterized mothers of toddlers who later were in need of short-term mental health services more often as "matter-of-fact" (38 percent vs. 23 percent) and "easy-going" (32 percent vs. 20 percent) and described control mothers more often as "affectionate" (45 percent vs. 23 percent).

There were no significant differences between future SMH children and controls in the psychologists' ratings of their intellectual and psychological status or in mean scores on the Cattell Infant Intelligence Scale, which fell in the normal range for both groups (96.0 for SMH; 99.6 for controls). There were also no significant differences between the two groups of toddlers on the pediatricians' ratings of physical development at age 2.

The only significant difference that emerged from our analysis of the data in early childhood was a difference on the Vineland Social Maturity Scale (Doll 1953), a measure of social competence. Toddlers who later were found to be in need of short-term mental health services had lower mean social quotients than controls on this scale—the differences appeared mostly in the areas of self-help, self-direction, and socialization (mean for SMH=114; mean for controls=120; $p < .05$).

In sum, there emerges an early picture of a group of infants without major biological impairment but who are somewhat dependent and socially immature as toddlers and whose needs in early childhood appear to be met by well-meaning but childlike and easygoing mothers who may not be too resourceful.

The Home at Ages 2 and 10

There were no significant differences between future SMH children and controls in ratings of family stability at age 2: Only 5 percent of future SMH and none of the control children came from homes rated low or very low in family stability. By the time these children had reached age 10, however, there was a significant difference between the two groups in ratings of emotional support in the home. Three out of four (74 percent) of the children considered in need of short-term mental health services at age 10 came from homes rated low (52 percent) or very low (22 percent) in emotional support, in contrast to less than one out of three (30.4 percent) of the control children (chi square=22.14, df=2;

$p < .001$). There was no significant difference between children in need of short-term mental health services and controls on ratings of educational stimulation provided by the home.

Contact with Community Agencies during Adolescence

Table 15 summarizes results of agency contacts of SMH children and controls for the eight-year period between ages 10 and 18. As can be seen from Table 15, there were some significant differences in agency contacts between SMH youth and controls without problems. Differences were significant for the total rate of agency contacts ($p < .001$), for rates of contact with Family Court and police ($p < .02$), and with the Division of Public Welfare ($p < .02$). However, the overall rate of agency contacts for SMH youth (43 percent) did not differ from that for the 1955 cohort (42 percent) and was much lower than that of the youth in need of long-term mental health services (76 percent) or those in need of placement in learning disability classes (81 percent). Less than half of all SMH youth, 4 out of 10 (the rate of the "unimproved" by age 18), had any contact with community agencies for problems that were much less serious than those of the LMH or LD youth.

Table 15   Differences in Agency Contacts Between SMH Youth and Matched Controls

Agency	SMH Youth (%) (N=60)	Controls (%) (N=60)	Chi Square*	p
Police	17.0	2.0	6.41	.02
Family Court	8.5	0	3.34	NS
Department of Health				
Public Health Nursing	7.0	2.0	.83	NS
Mental Health	5.0	0	1.37	NS
Department of Education				
Special Services	7.0	0	2.33	NS
High school counselors	10.0	2.0	2.43	NS
Department of Social Services				
Public Welfare (nonfinancial)	12.0	0	5.46	.02
Vocational Rehabilitation	3.0	0	.51	NS
Kauai hospitals†				
Teenage pregnancies	7.0	3.5	0	NS
Total with agency contacts	43.0	7.0	19.6	.001

* df=1.
† Females only.

The highest percentage of contacts (one out of six) was the police (17 percent); but the SMH cases had the lowest rate of repeaters (7 percent) of any of the problem groups and the smallest percentage of referrals to Family Court (8.5 percent). The most frequent offenses in this group were second-degree larceny and running away from home.

Only 1 out of 20 SMH youth (5 percent) had any contact with the Division of Mental Health between ages 10 and 18. They were seen for diagnostic workup only—without treatment. The diagnoses for the few cases that were seen by Mental Health did not contain any references to psychotic or neurotic or psychosomatic symptoms: Most were diagnosed as having adjustment reactions of adolescence or transient situational behavior disorders. Differences between SMH and LMH youth in contact with the Division of Mental Health were significant.

The Division of Public Welfare saw about one out of eight SMH cases (12 percent). Approximately 1 out of 10 became custody cases because of disturbed parent-child relationships, and 7 percent were placed in foster homes. Some girls came for pregnancy counseling, but the rate of illegitimate teenage pregnancies did not differ from the total rate for all 18-year-old women in the cohort. There were no abortions in this group. Differences between SMH and LMH youth in contact with the Division of Public Welfare were significant.

Group Test Results at Age 18

Although the children considered in need of short-term mental health services had scored within the normal range of intelligence on individual tests at ages 2 and 10 (mean Cattell IQ=96; mean PMA IQ=99), there were significant differences between them and the controls on all SCAT subtests in grade 12 and on the STEP reading and writing scales (see Table 16). There were also significant differences between the two groups on five subscales of the CPI. Three of the scales were measures of socialization; two were measures of achievement potential and intellectual efficiency.

Youth who needed short-term health services at age 10 scored significantly lower than their controls at age 18 on:

Responsibility ($p < .01$): identifies persons of conscientious, responsible, and dependable disposition

Socialization ($p < .02$): indicates the degree of social maturity, integrity, and rectitude the person has obtained

Achievement via independence ($p < .05$): identifies those factors of interest and motivation which facilitate achievement in any setting where autonomy and independence are positive behaviors

Intellectual efficiency ($p < .05$): indicates the degree of personal and intellectual efficiency the person has obtained

In contrast, they scored higher than controls on the good impression scale, which indicates a persistent concern about how others react to them ($p < .05$). Because the dimensions of the CPI are intercorrelated, a discriminant function analysis was run between the SMH and control groups. The same subscales separated the two groups to a significant extent.

Interview Results at Age 18

We were able to interview 49 (82 percent) of the youth who at age 10 had been considered in need of short-term mental health ser-

Table 16   Means and Standard Deviations on SCAT, STEP, and CPI Subscales Which Differentiated Significantly Between SMH Youth and Matched Controls at Age 18

Scale	SMH Youth (N=39)		Controls (N=39)		t	p
	Mean	SD	Mean	SD		
SCAT						
Verbal	26.5	23.3	44.9	23.8	3.30	<.01
Quantitative	32.6	27.2	46.5	26.2	2.19	<.05
Total	27.5	25.1	45.7	24.7	3.08	<.01
STEP						
Reading	29.5	26.8	46.8	25.9	2.88	<.01
Writing	32.9	25.4	28.9	23.7	2.78	<.01
CPI scales*						
Responsibility	20.7	3.8	24.2	5.2	3.29	<.01
Socialization	31.4	6.4	35.1	6.0	2.50	<.02
Good impression	13.4	4.5	11.2	4.9	1.97	<.05
Achievement via independence	12.6	3.6	14.6	3.5	2.33	<.05
Intellectual efficiency	26.4	5.5	29.3	6.3	2.04	<.05

* N=39 for SMH youth; N=32 for controls.

Table 17   Interview Ratings of SMH Youth at Age 18

Dimension	All SMH Interviewed (%) (N=44)	Untreated SMH Interviewed (%) (N=41)
Overall attitude toward school		
(very) favorable	55	54
mixed reactions	30	29
(very) unfavorable	16	17
Achievement motivation		
(very) high	52	49
content to get by	32	36
(very) low	16	15
Participation in school activities		
(very) extensive	20	19
some	32	32
(very) limited	48	49
Realism of educational plans beyond high school		
(very) realistic	75	78
mixed elements	20	19
(very) unrealistic	5	3
Job satisfaction		
(very) satisfied	72	70
ambivalent	17	18
(very) dissatisfied	11	12
Social life		
(very) good	61	63
fair	29	27
(very) poor	10	10
Feeling of security as part of family		
(very) strong	63	63
fair	20	20
(very) weak	16	17
Identification with mother		
identifies (strongly)	75	73
in conflict	11	15
(very) rejecting	14	12
Identification with father		
identifies (strongly)	64	66
in conflict	16	19
(very) rejecting	20	15
Overall family adjustment		
(very) good	50	56
fair	32	24
(very) poor	18	20
Degree of self-insight		
(very) high	32	34
some	36	37

Table 17 (Continued)

Dimension	All SMH Interviewed (%) (N=44)	Untreated SMH Interviewed (%) (N=41)
little or none	32	29
Extent of goal and value differentiation		
(very) great	42	44
some	23	22
little or none	35	34
Intensity of conflict feelings		
(very) great	14	12
some	45	46
little or none	41	41
Self-esteem		
(very) high	45	49
fair	34	29
(very) low	21	22

vices. As can be seen from Table 17, the majority of those interviewed (none of whom had received any mental health services since age 10) had made a satisfactory adjustment by age 18.

Though participation in school activities had been very limited for most during their high school days, the majority of the SMH youth had now a favorable overall attitude toward school and three out of four had realistic educational plans beyond high school. Their present favorable overall attitude toward school was exemplified by comments like these: "Good—pretty good—you need education. . . . It was good. [*Question*] Was fun most of all, you get to see all your friends, but I did kind of good and it was important to do well." . . . "It was all right. . . . This year I really did great . . . brought up all my grades so it was worthwhile this year. . . . I found I could really do something." And: "Oh, I loved it when I was a senior, wanted to be a freshman again. . . . Maybe some hard times, but good on the whole. . . . First it wasn't so very important to do well, I figured next year I can do better, finally saw this is it, no more next year, so I settled down."

In comparison with those who had been considered in need of long-term mental health services at age 10, more SMH youth planned to go to college (45 percent of SMH vs. 35 percent of LMH) and more had definite vocational plans (60 percent of SMH vs. 33

percent of LMH). Of those working, three out of four were satisfied with their jobs and nearly two out of three considered their present social life very satisfactory. One-third of the SMH youth were not living with their natural parents at the time of the 18-year interview, but two out of three expressed a very strong feeling of security as part of their family. Comments indicative of their present strong feeling of security as part of their family were: "I get along good with my parents . . . feel pretty close to mother and close to father too. . . . They understand me good . . . know everything what I do." And another youth: "We are close, I guess, we talk to each other. I tell my mother my problems. . . . Same thing with my father, only a little less. . . . They understand pretty well." And from another: "My mother's wonderful . . . I love her! [*Father*?] He's grumpy but isn't that a father for you? I like him too . . . guess raising a girl is hard. . . . We get along very good, though I'm closer to mother. . . . They understand enough to see my point." And: "My father? He's OK. He's cool . . . we get along pretty good. I'd say they understand me good enough."

Four out of five identified strongly with their mother, and two out of three with their father. Only about one out of three was rated by the interviewer as having little or no self-insight and little or no goal and value differentiation. Only about one out of five was rated as having a low self-esteem at age 18. Asked to describe themselves, they commented: "Once you get to know me I think I'm a friendly person. On the surface I try to be cool and let other people show their identity before I show myself. I think I'm helpful to other people. . . . I think I'm very complicated. . . . On the whole I'm pleased." And another remarked: "I'm an average everyday person. . . . I'll try to make a living." And another: "I don't know about me . . . I'm all right, I guess. Sometimes happy. I'm happy and unhappy as a person. . . . I'd like to see some changes. [*Question*] Kinda hard to say what." And another: "I don't think nothing of myself. I don't like to tell you I'm nice like that—it's up to a guy to find out how I am."

Only approximately 1 out of 10 of the SMH youth saw a need for psychotherapy during adolescence because of lack of self-confidence, "bad temper," or poor school performance. In contrast, 4 out of 10 of the LMH youth considered psychotherapy in adolescence.

Only 1 out of 10 among the SMH youth received any help by community agencies during adolescence, the smallest proportion among any of the groups of youth at risk. Four were counseled, four were placed in a foster home, and two were placed in the Job Corps. One youth, the most seriously disturbed in the group, was committed to the Hawaii State Mental Hospital by the Family Court but has since been released.

The overwhelming majority of the SMH youth received help from nonprofessional sources and considered this help effective. Peer friends (36.4 percent), older friends (31.8 percent), and parents (22.7 percent) were among the most frequently mentioned. School counselors (18.2 percent), teachers (6.8 percent), ministers (6.8 percent), and other professionals (2.3 percent) were less often mentioned. However, only one out of three among the SMH youth considered peer friends as the main source of help, in comparison with two out of three among the LMH youth (36 percent vs. 67 percent; $p < .10$). Fortunately, of all the groups of youth at risk, those in need of short-term mental health services had the highest improvement rate. Even among those who did not receive any help from community agencies, 60 percent were judged to be improved by the time they were 18 years old.

With few exceptions (3 out of 24) the improved cases had all been troubled by lack of self-confidence, anxiety, or chronic nervous habits in middle childhood. Among the 40 percent whose status had remained unchanged or who had deteriorated since age 10 were most of the children (13 out of 16) who had been characterized by anxiety and acting-out problems in the elementary grades. (See Chapter 10.)

Discussion

As a group, the children who needed only short-term mental health services at age 10 appear to have a more favorable prognosis than their contemporaries with learning disabilities and long-term mental health needs. Most were free of biological impairment at birth and did not suffer from serious impairment in infant-mother attachment before age 2. Though most came from poor homes socioeconomically, their families were relatively stable throughout their early childhood.

There is a hint, however, from the results of our two-year developmental examinations that these children, as toddlers, were less socially mature and more dependent than control children of the same sex, and socioeconomic and ethnic background and that their mothers were somewhat childlike and easygoing as parents.

By the time these children had reached age 10, their dependency and lack of self-confidence had become aggravated by a home situation that now gave little of the emotional support they needed. In addition, a significant proportion had developed minor and moderate physical handicaps (25 percent of SMH vs. 2 percent of controls; chi square=11.25, df=1; $p < .001$). They were now shy and anxious. Many had developed chronic nervous habits and reverted to behavior immature for their age to deal with their insecurities. Though they scored within the normal range of intelligence on individual tests at ages 2 and 10, they did poorly on group tests requiring communication skills and were recognized as having behavior problems by their teachers in the early elementary grades. Eight years later, however, at the threshold of young adulthood, the status of the majority of these children has considerably improved, though very few in this group (only 1 in about 10) had received any positive help from community agencies and none the mental health services recommended by the panel and suggested in a letter to their parents.

To be sure, there were still some residual problems, especially in social and achievement behavior, at age 18. Their response to a self-report inventory showed them to be still somewhat socially immature and unwilling to accept responsibility. In comparison with contemporaries who had no problems at age 10, they appeared more handicapped in situations where autonomy and independence were valued. As a group, they were still unable to make the most efficient use of their intellectual potential. They were concerned and sensitive about how others reacted to them, and there was a tendency for them to want to create a good impression on people in authority. A sizable proportion (45 percent) wanted to change some of their personality traits and considered lack of self-confidence, bad temper, and poor scholarship among their weak points.

Few in this group, however, had become serious mental health problems or problems to the community during the turbulent years of adolescence. Delinquency rates and rates of illegitimate teenage pregnancies were lower for this group than any of the other groups of youth at risk and comparable to those of the 1955 cohort. Not only were their infringements less frequent, they were also of a less serious nature and less repetitive.

A smaller proportion of this group than of any of the other problem groups had presented serious discipline or learning problems in school, and even the few who were referred to mental health services had not developed any serious psychosomatic, neurotic, or psychotic symptoms (with the exception of one boy referred by the Family Court to a state mental hospital because of problems with sexual identity).

By age 18, the majority of the teenagers who at age 10 had been considered in need of short-term mental health services had a good social and family life, were satisfied with their jobs, and, if not working, had realistic educational plans that for many included college. About one-third no longer lived with both natural parents, but the majority felt secure as part of their family. Most identified with their mothers, and the majority with their fathers. Only about a third were rated as having little self-insight and goal and value differentiation. Only about 1 in 10 had intense conflict feelings and saw a need for psychotherapy. Most encouraging was the high improvement rate among children considered in need of short-term mental health services at age 10. By age 18, some 60 percent were judged to be improved.

This improvement rate in our multiracial group of youth on Kauai is identical with the rate in a population of Caucasian children in England. Of all the follow-up studies of childhood behavior problems reviewed (see Table 3), this British study comes closest to ours in design. It is based on a countywide survey of grade school children whose behavior problems were identified by maternal interviews and teachers' behavior checklists. These children had received no treatment by the time of the follow-up in midadolescence. We are fortunate in having now both longitudinal and cross-cultural evidence that corroborates their findings that much of "behavior suggestive of emotional ill health in children tends to recede spontaneously in response to developmental changes or life circumstances" (Shepherd et al. 1971:162).

The degree to which peer friends, older friends, parents, and the gradual assumption of responsibilities (a job, moving away from home to get an education) have contributed to this improvement is best illustrated by excerpts from two of our interviews. One was with a young man, the other with a young woman, both of whom were among the youth who had short-term mental health problems in middle childhood but whose status improved without intervention by community agencies.

The young man had been described by his mother at 10 years as a child with occasional facial twitches, whose feelings were easily hurt and who had difficulties concentrating. He appeared restrained and constricted to the teacher, and his response to projective tests revealed to the psychologist "fantasies made up of a combination of yearning for simple affection and fear of retaliation for indiscretions." Excerpts from his 18-year interview follow:

> I: We've already talked a little bit about school, and now I'm interested in finding out what you're going to be doing in the future. . . . How far do you plan to go in school and college?
> S: I'd like to go to a four-year college. Right now I'm going to start out in a two-year college, and then transfer to a four-year college.
> I: Where are you going now?
> S: I'm going to Honolulu Community College and will transfer later to the University of Hawaii or somewhere.
> I: Do you have any idea what you want to take?
> S: I'm interested mainly in police science, criminology. [*Question*] I like to help people out. There's a lot to be done. [*Question*] I know a lot of relatives on the police force. [*Questioned about work*] I'm on the plantation this summer. I'll be in irrigation most of the summer. [*Question*] Yes, I worked in the pineapple fields for the past three years on Molokai.
> I: And what kind of things have been important to you when you were working?
> S: Getting along with others and learning to take orders from your supervisors.
> I: And what would be important in selecting a job in the future?
> S: Mainly the interest of the work. To find a job you're going to be interested in, you've got to like it. You don't want to work at a job that you're not interested in, I mean you don't enjoy it. I don't even care what the money is.

And about friends:

> I: How well do you think you get along with people?

S: The right people I get along with all right, but it depends. If they don't like me, then it's hard to get along with them.

I: Do you think most people like you?

S: I guess so. I don't see why they don't.

I: What kind of people do you not like to associate with?

S: People who are too bossy, or people who like to do things their way when there are other ways. I don't like those who push you into things that may get you into trouble.

I: And what kind of people do you look up to?

S: People who are friendly and like to do things that I do. I guess that's all.

And about his girlfriend:

S: We were going steady for a while, but I didn't want to be tied down. We're just friends. I just want to enjoy being by myself, see if I can handle it. [*After describing his parents favorably, he continues.*] We get along pretty well. When I have a problem or something, we can be open and I talk to them. I'm not afraid of them.

I: How close do you feel to your mother? Do you feel closer to your mother or father?

S: I think I have an equal relationship with them. I just love them both.

I: How well do you think they understand you?

S: I think they understand me. They should. All these years I've been open to them. They do pretty well when I need help or am in trouble. I don't get into trouble, but when I need help with a problem.

I: Parents influence their children in different ways. How do you think your mother has influenced you?

S: Just giving a good example. A lot of things I see in my family are different from other families. We always think of the family first, then friends.

I: And your father, how do you think he's influenced you?

S: I'm very happy I got a father like that. He likes to do outdoor stuff. Lots of boys don't get to enjoy things like that, fishing, diving. I guess my father is a jack of all trades. He likes to do all kinds of stuff—lots of sports.

I: What did your parents stress when you were growing up?

S: They always said to keep to my studies, to study well because they had a hard life and they don't want me to go through that stage that they went through. They always stress that I should learn a lot and find a job so I don't have to struggle. Be good in school, get a good education.

I: Did they say anything special they want you to be?

S: They just leave it up to me. They didn't push, they just leave it up to me and my interests.

I: Different families say different things are important. What kind of things did yours emphasize as being right?

S: They emphasized our love. I can't think of anything else. They taught that the family is first, then your friends. You always help out your family.

I: Have any other members of your family had a major influence on you, do you think?

S: I learned a lot from my older brother about what I should do. [*Question*] He's in Honolulu, finished two years of college and is working in an office.

And later:

I: Do you have any special goals or objectives that you're working towards?

S: Like I said, I'd like to finish up a four-year college and get a job, mainly in police work. I wanted to go into wildlife management, but academically I wasn't that good. I guess I'll take police work and try to get into law enforcement.

I: What do you think you really want to achieve out of life, what do you really look forward to and most want to get out of your life?

S: Happiness in everything I do, and I don't like to have problems. I see myself giving help to others who need help. Give advice to others and help them enjoy life and find a better way to live.

I: Everybody worries about something. What sort of things worry you?

S: Not being able to fulfill my goals. . . . I don't worry a lot. It's all up to me to do the things I want to do. [*Questioned about the most important experiences and influences that have helped make him the kind of person he is.*] Mainly my parents and my friends.

The second subject, a female, sucked her thumb until age 7, had a history of severe tantrums, was easily hurt, and had frequent crying spells and headaches. At 18 years she said:

S: Most of all I just like to enjoy life. [*Questioned about how she felt about high school.*] My freshman year, naturally I was scared and the years went by and I got used to school, you know, it was like my second home in a way. Like every student, I had a teacher I hated, well, not hated, but I didn't get along with. Just the other day I was driving past thinking, hey, I'm going to miss this school. I'm going to Honolulu for school and I won't be able to be here, see my teachers or friends. [*Questioned about how well she'd done and her plans.*] My other years I didn't do all that well, but then I started buckling down. I made the honor roll through my senior year all the way. . . . I plan to go to a two-year college, but at the end of my two years, when I graduate from there, I might change my mind and continue on in college. It all depends. I think I can make it.

I: Do you think when you're finished you will work, get married, or both?

S: I don't plan to get married until I'm about twenty-three, twenty-four maybe. I figure too many people get married too young and they don't really know what they're going into, and a lot of them end up if not divorced, then separated, like my brother and wife. They got married kind of young, and I don't want myself to be in that situation where you're always fighting. You should be mature and know what you're going into before you do anything. . . . I'll work after my kids are in school. If you leave them with a babysitter too long, it leaves the children with a sense of longing. A parent should be with the child until they're in school at least, so that when a child comes home, they won't be away from them that long. Because when they go to a babysitter every day and see the parents only a couple of hours a day, it's wrong. [*Questioned about friends.*] My boyfriend is seven years older than I am. We've been going together for about two years, but I feel that an older person is good for a woman—I don't know how to explain it. They are settled, they're not the flighty type. We don't have any serious plans until I'm older. He knows that I have to continue school and wait awhile and pay my loan off.

I: How well do you think you get along with people?

S: Very well. Well, I'm kind of shy before I get to know you, but once I get to know you, I don't want to brag but I'm really outgoing, and I like people. I think my personality is good enough for people to like me. I haven't lost friends. . . . I don't like to associate with people that think they're too good for others, you know. Just because I didn't have the money. Besides, you can tell when you're not liked, too, if you're different from others. I don't like people that think they're better than anybody else.

I: [*Questions her about her parents, what they are like, whether she is similar to them, how they get along.*]

S: My mother started going through the change of life early and I guess she's still kind of going through it. She doesn't always feel good, and everything sort of bothers her. I guess she's lonely too. . . . My father's very soft-hearted. Even though he didn't want

me to go to Honolulu or school, he won't stop me 'cause he wants
me to be happy, and he really cares for our happiness. . . . I'm like
my father. My father, if he has money or something, and he doesn't
need it and someone else needs it, he'll give it to them. That's the
way I am, I'm not selfish or anything. . . . When my mother's not
grumpy, I can talk to her in a mother-daughter way. If I have problems I can talk to her. But I'm a lot closer to my boyfriend's
mother. . . . Well, my father, we're really close, but he's Filipino
style, still old-fashioned in ways. They feel that I shouldn't grow up
like that. They are modern, but they're not really up to date, as
open-minded as people are nowadays. . . . My mother used to hit
me and beat me. That's how come I'm not very close to her. . . . I
used to hate my mother, but after awhile, as I got older, I under-
stood how she was going through that change of life. So I became a
little more understanding of her, but I really haven't gotten too close
to her. Mother and daughter really should be close to each other.
I'm closer to my father. He's made me decide what I want to do,
and he's always advised me, "Don't do anything unless you know
what you're doing." So he's the one that's influenced me about the
marriage part.

I: [*Questions her about herself, things she wants to change or
develop.*]

S: Well, in my first part of my high school years, I really had a hot
temper, but I've learned to control myself. I can control myself, but
I can take things only up to a point. I guess everybody's like that. I
try to think things out calmly and try to think of a solution to things.
Don't jump to conclusions. That's how I got excited a lot. I used to
race, and I really had a hot temper. I mean people would just say a
certain thing to me, and I'd just jump at them. But now I think
before I act. . . . I feel that I want to do something important, but I
don't know. . . . I guess maybe after I'm through school, maybe
something will happen. . . . I want to get the most out of life and
enjoy it, 'cause you never know what's going to happen the next
day. I take each day as it comes and enjoy it. . . . I'm going to live
each day as it comes along.

I: [*Questions her about worries, problems.*]

S: I always worry if someone is going to like me when I first meet
them, but after I get to know them and they get to know me, then I
don't think about things like that. But everybody is self-conscious
about their appearance, I guess, about their actions, or if someone
will like them. I guess it's a natural feeling. I used to worry that I
was going to die the next day. That was when I was younger
though. . . . I was too embarrassed to talk to counselors at school,

but I talk to my boyfriend's mother a lot about certain problems and she advised me pretty well. And my boyfriend's sister. Actually, I'm pretty close to them.

I: What do you think are the most important experiences and influences that have helped make you the kind of person you are?

S: Well, I guess if my father had kept being strict with me and I kept sneaking out, I guess I may have turned out more the rugged type, you know. All the boys and girls in my family have all graduated from school and have been good, you know, so I guess I followed in their footsteps. I don't want to shame my family.

In sum, the prognosis for shy, anxious children with nervous habits, but without marked biological impairment and disturbed early mother-child relationships, appears much more favorable than for children with learning disabilities and those in need of long-term mental health services (especially the acting-out problems), many of whom appear to suffer from the cumulative effect of an impaired biological disposition and early affective deprivation. The resiliency of the human spirit is demonstrated in the fact that in most instances positive changes occurred without intervention. The significance of this for community planning for the delivery of services to children is discussed later in Chapter 14.

CHAPTER 8
New Problems in Adolescence

On the basis of records from the schools and other community agencies we identified 45 additional youths (30 females, 15 males) who had developed serious behavior problems in adolescence. The ratio of girls to boys in this group was 2:1. Among them were 23 teenage pregnancies. The other five pregnant teenagers were among the cases of learning disabilities and mental health problems already identified at age 10. Among the new problems were also 19 youths who had been in trouble with the law. The other 139 delinquents in this age group were among those who had been considered in need of remedial education, special class placement, or mental health services at age 10. Finally, there were two youths who had made suicide attempts during adolescence and two who had dropped out of high school before graduation.

Contact with Community Agencies during Adolescence

As can be seen in Table 18, this group, during adolescence, had a rate of contact with the Family Court that was five times as high as that of their peers in the 1955 cohort, a rate of contact with their high school counselors that was four times as high, and a rate of contact with the Divisions of Mental Health and Public Welfare that was three times as high.

Of the major ethnic groups in the community, youth of Hawaiian and part-Hawaiian descent were overrepresented

Table 18 Rates of Agency Contacts During Adolescence for New Problems and Total 1955 Cohort

Agency	New Problems (%) (N=45)	1955 Cohort (%) (N=696)
Police	70.0	23.0
Family Court	35.0	7.0
Department of Health		
Public Health Nursing	7.0	7.0
Mental Health	12.0	4.0
Department of Education		
Special Services	10.0	8.0
High school counselors	37.0	9.0
Department of Social Services		
Public Welfare	37.0	14.0
Vocational Rehabilitation	2.5	2.0
Kauai hospitals*		
Teenage pregnancies	70.0	8.0

* Females only.

among the new problems in adolescence (43 percent vs. 22 percent in the 1955 cohort) and youth of Japanese descent were under-represented (15 percent vs. 33 percent in the 1955 cohort), as they had been among the cases of learning disabilities and mental health problems identified in childhood.

An inspection of our earlier data reveals no significant differences between the new problem cases and control cases of the same age and sex without problems at age 10 and 18 on *any* of the birth variables, on behavior and home observations in infancy, and on the results of the physical and psychological examinations during the 2-year and 10-year follow-up. This group of youth had scored within the normal range of intelligence on developmental tests at age 2 and on group tests of ability at age 10 and had not had a disproportionate need for short- or long-term remedial educational help in grades 1 to 5. However, a high proportion of youth who developed serious behavior problems in adolescence came from homes rated low (45 percent) and very low (29 percent) in socioeconomic status and low (43 percent) or very low (29 percent) in educational stimulation at age 10. By comparison, only 12 percent of the 1955 cohort had been rated very low in SES and only 11 percent were very low in educational stimulation provided in the home.

Group Test Results at Age 18

Consistent with our findings at age 10, mean scores of the new problem group on the SCAT and the STEP did not differ significantly from the "complement group," those of the 1955 cohort without problems.

There was a tendency, however, for the new problem cases to score in the external direction on the Novicki Locus of Control Scale. These differences (see Table 19) were statistically significant for the teenage pregnancies among them (mean scores for pregnant teenagers=15.7, those for controls of same age and sex=13.0; $p < .05$). As a group, these youth believed that events happened to them as a result of fate or other factors beyond their control. There were also a number of dimensions on the CPI that differentiated significantly between new problem cases in adolescence and controls of the same age and sex who had no behavior problems at 10 or 18. Differences were apparent on measures of self-assurance (capacity for status and social presence), socialization, responsibility, achievement potential, intellectual efficiency, and flexibility (see Table 20).

As a group, the new problem cases in adolescence scored significantly lower than controls of the same age and sex on the following dimensions:

1. Capacity for status: assesses the qualities that lead to status
2. Responsibility: identifies persons of conscientious, responsible, and dependable behavior
3. Socialization: indicates the degree of social maturity, integrity, and rectitude the person has attained
4. Achievement via conformance: measures factors of interest and motivation that facilitate achievement in which conformance is positive behavior
5. Intellectual efficiency: indicates the degree of personal and intellectual efficiency the person has attained
6. Flexibility: assesses the degree of flexibility and adaptability of the person's thinking and social behavior

As a group the adolescent problem cases appeared to be restricted in outlook and interests; uneasy and awkward in unfamiliar social situations; immature, undercontrolled, and impulsive in behavior; defensive, headstrong, and rebellious; easily disorganized under stress or pressure to conform; lacking in self-direction and self-discipline; and worrying and guarded.

As one of them said: "I gotta take the burn. Right now I see this a ripped out world . . . only way can make out is by burning or ripping out. I'm no exception." And another: "I wanted to do the same things and go to the same places as my brother but was never good enough. . . . I feel I'm sick of school. Maybe I might try technical college later on but no decision yet. . . . I want to cruise for a year and then decide. [*What do you want to achieve out of life?*] Enjoyment. [*Question*] Having fun . . . doing whatever I want to do." A third expressed some concern: "Right now I don't know what I'm going to do when I grow up and graduate. I'm getting worried now—pretty soon I'll have to be on my own."

On a number of additional CPI dimensions, the teenage pregnancies among the new problems differed from other young women in the 1955 cohort who were not pregnant. They scored significantly lower than controls of the same age and sex on:

1. Social presence: assesses factors such as poise, spontaneity, and self-confidence in personal and social interaction
2. Tolerance: identifies persons with permissive, accepting, and nonjudgmental social beliefs and attitudes
3. Achievement via independence: measures those factors of interest and motivation that facilitate achievement in settings where autonomy and independence are positive behaviors

Thus, in contrast to the stereotyped image of the popular girl, most teenagers who were pregnant during adolescence lacked poise, spontaneity, and self-confidence in personal and social situations. They were aloof, wary, and retiring; they were distrustful in personal and social outlook; they were anxious and lacking in self-insight and self-understanding. Their interview responses tend to confirm the picture revealed on the CPI:

I never was the kind to stay with a lot of friends. I'd end up picking the wrong kind, get into trouble. . . . The only person I went out with was my boyfriend.

I know I missed a lot in high school as I never really cared about studies. I messed around. Now I really regret it.

I'm unhappy. I always wished I was dead.

I don't think the teachers like me. [*Question*] Pick on me . . . I'm not satisfied. I wish I could be born again and start all over.

Table 19 Significant Differences Between Pregnant Teenagers and Nonpregnant Controls of Same Age on CPI and Locus of Control Scale

Scale	Teenage Pregnancies (N=15)		Control Females (N=152)		t	p
	Mean	SD	Mean	SD		
California Psychological Inventory						
Capacity for status	11.27	2.96	13.61	3.62	2.85	.01
Social presence	28.27	4.38	30.77	5.18	2.07	.05
Responsibility	18.80	5.99	24.33	5.49	3.43	.003
Socialization	28.00	5.89	34.57	6.06	4.11	.001
Tolerance	10.33	4.64	13.39	5.08	2.42	.02
Achievement via conformance	16.80	4.04	20.71	4.96	3.50	.003
Achievement via independence	11.40	3.74	13.83	4.02	2.38	.02
Intellectual efficiency	23.53	5.22	28.44	6.04	3.42	.003
Flexibility	6.00	3.38	7.93	3.68	2.09	.05
Novicki Locus of Control*	15.69	4.52	13.07	4.42	2.01	.04

* N=13 for teenage pregnancies; N=151 for controls.

Table 20 Means and Standard Deviations on CPI Subscales Which Differentiated Significantly Between New Problems at Age 18 and Controls of Same Age and Sex without Problems

CPI Scale	New Problems (N=26)		Controls (N=273)		t	p
	Mean	SD	Mean	SD		
Capacity for status	11.7	3.2	13.6	3.6	2.57	.01
Responsibility	20.3	6.3	23.3	5.1	2.19	.05
Socialization	28.3	6.7	33.2	6.5	3.17	.001
Achievement via conformance	16.2	4.4	20.0	4.7	3.74	.001
Intellectual efficiency	24.5	6.7	27.9	6.0	2.45	.02
Flexibility	6.8	3.1	8.3	3.6	2.04	.05

I got one special friend, but to me I don't think people like me much, but I like them.

How would I describe myself? Rotten! [*Laughs*] No, I don't know.

Interview Results at Age 18

We were able to interview 41 (91 percent) of the 45 new problem cases, among them all teenage pregnancies, all suicide attempts, all school dropouts, and all but four of the delinquents. As can be seen from Table 21, the majority of the youth in this group had, at the threshold of adulthood, persistent problems in their social and family life and reported intense conflict feelings accompanied by little self-insight and low self-esteem. Interview ratings that were made without any knowledge of the public record or their responses to self-report inventories confirmed the picture that emerged from the California Psychological Inventory.

Nearly three out of four in this group (70 percent) had been limited in their participation in school activities, and only one out of three (35 percent) was judged to have a satisfactory social life upon leaving high school. While the majority (75 percent) of those working were satisfied with their jobs, one out of two (52 percent) had mixed to unrealistic plans for the future and two out of three (62 percent) were either rated as "content to get by" or low in achievement motivation. Only about half (54 percent) had a favorable attitude toward their school experience and more than half (56 percent) had only limited goals for the future.

Table 21   Differences Between Treated and Untreated New Problems at Age 18 on Interview Ratings

Dimension	Total (%) (N=41)	Treated (%) (N=10)	Untreated (%) (N=31)	p*
Overall attitude toward school				
(very) favorable	54.0	30	59	.09
mixed reactions	27.0	30	28	
(very) unfavorable	19.0	40	13	
Achievement motivation				
(very) high	38.0	10	45	.06
content to get by	49.0	80	45	
(very) low	13.0	10	10	
Participation in school activities				
(very) extensive	8.0	0	13	.19
some	22.0	20	24	
(very) limited	70.0	80	63	

Table 21   (Continued)

Dimension	Total (%) (N=41)	Treated (%) (N=10)	Untreated (%) (N=31)	p*
Realism of educational plans beyond high school				
(very) realistic	48.0	30	52	.67
mixed elements	46.0	50	45	
(very) unrealistic	6.0	20	3	
Job satisfaction				
(very) satisfied	75.0	50	80	.41
ambivalent	17.0	0	20	
(very) dissatisfied	8.0	50	—	
Social life				
(very) good	35.0	10	45	.05
fair	49.0	80	41	
(very) poor	16.0	10	14	
Feeling of security as part of family				
(very) strong	38.0	30	30	.31
fair	38.0	30	35	
(very) weak	24.0	40	35	
Identification with mother				
identifies (strongly)	56.0	50	48	.28
in conflict	14.0	20	21	
(very) rejecting	30.0	30	31	
Identification with father				
identifies (strongly)	54.0	30	45	.22
in conflict	24.0	40	27.5	
(very) rejecting	22.0	30	27.5	
Overall family adjustment				
(very) good	27.0	0	31	.05
fair	38.0	50	21	
(very) poor	35.0	50	48	
Degree of self-insight				
(very) high	32.0	20	41	.15
some	57.0	60	52	
little or none	11.0	20	7	
Extent of goal and value differentiation				
(very) great	44.0	20	52	.07
some	31.0	50	17	
little	25.0	30	31	
Intensity of conflict feelings				
(very) great	47.0	80	52	.09
some	39.0	10	31	
little	14.0	10	17	
Self-esteem				
high	22.0	10	24	.03
fair	47.0	30	55	
(very) low	31.0	60	21	

* Fisher's exact probability test.

At the threshold of adulthood, they appeared to derive little support from their families: "My mother? Well now, she's a housewife. She cares for us but not when I was there—used to drink—better now as she has ulcers. But when she drank, she razed me down for nothing. So I went out and got into trouble." Another, questioned about how close she felt to her mother, said: "I don't know. I can't describe that kind of stuff." Questioned about her father: "Not too close—I didn't get along with my parents. I guess I was trying to get even with them for doing something. I didn't know what they did."

Only about one out of four (27 percent) had a satisfactory family adjustment by age 18, and only about one out of three (38 percent) felt secure as part of their family. Nearly one out of two were in conflict with or rejected their father (46 percent) or their mother (44 percent). A similar proportion (47 percent) had intense conflict feelings. In the words of one:

> I just walk away when my father sees me. I don't feel close to him, nothing to say to him. . . . Y'know, I *wish* I'd get a scolding from my father. Y'know, the past Christmas I come home at one-thirty or two. He asked how come I come home late, but no scolding. If I got scolding, I would listen.

And still another:

> To me my mother is emotionally sick—and the doctor has said it. . . . She's sick, she knows it, picks on us and father. . . . I don't feel any closeness, don't have that close feeling. [*Question*] I guess the same with my father, just at times, don't know why I sense a difference. [*Question*] They don't understand me at all . . . but I worry a lot about my family. I want to help. [*Later*] But I want to shut out what bothers me and just keep to myself now.

Bad temper, willfulness, weakness, and lack of self-confidence were recognized by them most frequently as their weak points. Two out of three (68 percent) had little self-insight and nearly a third (31 percent) were rated low in self-esteem. A third of this group of youth saw the need for some outside help; the others never thought of it, or considered it but did not go. One of the teenage pregnancies reported:

> I never saw a doctor till the day of birth—had no help, I just went to friends and found out in the books. My parents found out one day before I gave birth. I lied to them, I'm naturally fat and told them I

was coming fat. I never told my boyfriend till he came back. I was one and a half months *hapai* ["pregnant"] when he left. . . . I didn't know the public health nurse then, but now I do, and I got help later.

One out of every three new problem cases (15 out of 45) did receive some positive intervention from community agencies: 13 were counseled through the police, Family Court, or high school; 3 had been hospitalized and received individual, group, or drug therapy; 3 had been aided by Big Sister volunteers; 3 had been placed in foster homes; and 3 were tutored at home during their pregnancies.

A higher proportion among the new problems in adolescence turned to counselors (19 percent) and professionals (22 percent) for help than among those whose problems were identified in childhood. As with all other problem youth, peer friends were the most frequent source of help cited (32 percent). Older friends (13.5 percent) and parents (5 percent) were much less frequently mentioned as sources of help than among those with childhood behavior problems. None in this group had gone to a teacher or minister for help.

In general, the new problem cases were about evenly divided between those who thought they had been helped by outside assistance and those who thought it was of little or no help to them. One reported:

I went to the school counselor about my pregnancy. I didn't know what to do. We considered abortion as we were afraid of my parents, but we really wanted this baby. [*Question*] Afraid that it would really put them [parents] down and embarrass them—but we really wanted it bad as we wouldn't do it [sex] if we didn't love each other. Parents are happy now and proud of the baby. [*Question*] My boyfriend and I saw him [counselor] a lot. We used to go down to church and he'd come over and talk to us. . . . It was really good talking to him.

But another said:

I asked for help and got the runaround. . . . I went in a couple times and the lady came to see me, said she'd come back tomorrow and never showed up.

A comparison of interview ratings between the new problem cases who had received some positive agency intervention and those who had not (see Table 21) revealed some significant differences ($p < .05$): Among the treated new problem cases was a higher proportion with a poor social and family life than among the untreated and a higher proportion of youth with low self-esteem. In general, intervention by community agencies during adolescence went to those worse off (see Chapter 9).

Among the cases of learning disabilities and mental health problems identified at age 10, there were no significant sex and socioeconomic differences between those who received some form of positive intervention by community agencies and those who did not. Among the new problems in adolescence, however, a higher proportion of boys than girls were assisted by community agencies. One might speculate that the boys may have gotten more attention because of the nuisance value of their delinquent acts. That the adolescent girls in this group need the community's help desperately is evident from the interview responses of the pregnant teenagers (only 10 percent of whom received any outside help).

In contrast to the positive anticipation of the future that characterized most interviews among the nonpregnant control women in the 1955 cohort, the responses of the pregnant teenagers told a depressing tale of lack of opportunities, lack of close friends and confidants, lack of parental support and understanding, lack of faith in the efficacy of one's own effort, and, most of all, lack of self-esteem (see Tables 22 and 23). The following case of a pregnant teenager reveals much of this pattern:

> **Case A. C.:** The middle child of 13, this girl became known to the police at age 17 as a runaway and for larceny. By age 18 she was living with her boyfriend, and school reports indicated poor attendance but said she would probably graduate. Interviewed in the fall following her graduation and marriage, she indicated that she had missed a lot in high school and regretted it now: "I put my schooling aside and wanted to be free. I used to be really mixed up." She had moved out of her home as "mother kept picking on me and beating me up—accused me of being interested in boys and I wasn't." She had gone with her boyfriend for three years, "never got love from anyone else."
>
> Questioned about her parents, she said: "I hate to say—you won't tell her? She's two-faced, can't trust her.

She's the boss and dad can't stand up against her. I know she struggled a lot for us, and we really gave her one sickness that stays inside her . . . but I can't forget, never got anything. My dad? I just love my dad. He was so quiet and always had time to listen to me, was the only person I could talk to, but he didn't influence me at all—only my mom beating me up. But he spent most of his time working, earning money to support us. We had lots of bills, lots of kids. I worry about my brothers and sisters. . . . Now I worry about food rates, if I'll have a hard time to support my child."

She reported sniffing glue and smoking marijuana from grades 7 to 9 and said she "took dope" because of problems with her parents, adding: "But I felt I was pretty hooked on it, always needed it, so gradually I stopped—it was really amazing I stopped. But I was having bum trips—it brought back my past life."

Describing herself, she said: "I get hurt easily, I like to be treated soft, not mean. I'm bossy but I try not to be. I'm

Table 22   Significant Differences Between Teenage Pregnancies and Controls of Same Age on 18-Year Interview Ratings

Dimension	Teenage Pregnancies (%) (N=22)	Control Females (%) (N=23)	p*
Achievement motivation:			
Content to get by—(very) low	61	19	.009
Participation in school activities:			
(Very) limited	74	19	.0008
Realism of educational plans beyond high school:			
Mixed—unrealistic	59	6	.0008
Identification with mother:			
In conflict—(very) rejecting	45	6	.009
Identification with father:			
In conflict—(very) rejecting	52	12	.01
Overall family adjustment:			
(Very) poor	35	6	.04
Goal and value differentiation:			
Fair—(very) low	56	12	.005
Self-esteem:			
Fair—(very) low	77	31	.02

* Fisher's exact probability test.

Table 23   Significant Differences Between Teenage Pregnancies
           and Controls of Same Age on 18-Year Interview Questions

Interview Questions	Teenage Pregnancies (%) (N=23)	Control Females (%) (N=23)	p*
Interests and activities:			
School organizations	22	75	.001
Educational plans:			
High school or less	52	19	.03
Career-marriage combination:			
Plans to marry, may work to earn money, but not interested in job or career	56	19	.03
Timing: work-marriage-parenthood:			
will work irrespective of age of children; will work, does not want children	59	19	.01
Definitiveness of vocational plans:			
Definite	35	81	.004
Vocation considered:			
Undecided	20	0	.03
Feature of job deemed important:			
Opportunity to use abilities	4	31	.03
Satisfaction with educational achievement:			
Doing well, proud of it	30	73	.004
Importance of doing well in school:			
High	13	69	.0003
Relationship with opposite sex:			
Married	48	0	.008
Makeup of nuclear family:			
Living with both natural parents	48	94	.02
View of mother as model:			
Would like all or some of her attributes	67	94	.05
Description of mother:			
(Mostly) positive	46	88	.008
Parents easy to talk to:			
Mother: most, all of the time	48	80	.001
Father: never, infrequently	55	7	.03
Parental goals for child:			
Father: moral, behavioral ("be good")	17	63	.005
Mother: moral, behavioral ("be good")	21	50	.03
Degree father has influenced child:			
None or little	48	12	.02
Disagreements in family:			
No resolution; argue, go separate ways	59	19	.02
Family talks together :			
Little	52	12	.01
Moral issues:			
Drugs, sex, "not getting in trouble"	60	28	.05
Subject of family rules:			
Letting parents know whereabouts	14	47	.03

Table 23 (Continued)

Interview Questions	Teenage Pregnancies (%) (N=23)	Control Females (%) (N=23)	p*
View of parental control:			
Father enforces rules consistently	0	31	.02
View of parental achievement demands:			
Father: college	0	50	.002
Mother: college	6	38	.03
View of parental support:			
Father: opposes, disagrees, uninterested	35	6	.04
Mother: opposes, disagrees, uninterested	43	6	.01
Strong points:			
Understanding, good listener	0	31	.01
Academic abilities	0	25	.03
Future goals:			
Social concern, close relation with others	4	31	.03
Worries:			
Some—much	87	38	.002
Kind of worry:			
Money	45	6	.009
Psychotherapy:			
Never thought of it	46	94	.001
Considered it, did not go	36	6	.03
Goes occasionally, regularly	18	0	.01
Sources of help:			
Older friends	17	50	.04
Professionals	26	0	.04

* Fisher's exact probability test.

really scared to say anything." She felt premarital sex to be "wrong, but at the rate the world's going on today, you have to try to find what you really want. I felt it was wrong to do, but I loved him so much I wanted to show him I loved him in that special way so I made love to him. . . . Nowadays all kids like it, just that good feeling, no shame to them. Guess they'll realize their mistakes as they grow older."

In contrast to the control women, the majority of pregnant teenagers had been content "to just get by" in high school and were rated very low in achievement motivation (61 percent vs. 19 percent). Few expressed any intrinsic satisfaction with their educational achievement (30 percent vs. 73 percent); even fewer thought it important to do well in school (13 percent vs. 69 percent). While in high school, participation in school activities and school-related organizations were very limited for most (74 percent vs. 19 percent). The majority did not plan to go beyond high school (52 percent), and none of their fathers and few (6 percent) of their mothers expected them to go on to college.

Educational and vocational plans beyond high school were mixed or unrealistic for most (59 percent). Only about a third (35 percent) had definite vocational plans, and very few (4 percent) were concerned about an opportunity to use their abilities. Most planned to marry—and to work to earn money—but were not interested in a job or career (56 percent). Most planned to work, irrespective of the age of their children (54 percent), and did not want any more children.

About half the pregnant teenagers were married; the other half were still living with both natural parents. Nearly half (45 percent) were in conflict with their fathers. Less than half (46 percent) described their mothers in positive tones or as "easy to talk to."

The majority (55 percent) never or only infrequently talked to their fathers, and about half (48 percent) felt that their fathers had little or no influence on them. Nearly half the pregnant teenagers felt that their fathers and mothers did not understand them and were unconcerned about them. More than a third felt that their parents opposed them, disagreed with them, or were uninterested in their ideas and plans.

The majority (52 percent) had families that talked little together, and there were no positive resolutions of disagreements among them. Most argued, then went their separate ways:

> We can't win against our parents, but there was lots of fighting in our family . . . bad hassles.

> It's a riot, a real riot—bad—but in an hour or two everyone is calming down and understanding each other.

> We argued, then somebody gets a licking. We just let it pass, no effort to resolve it.

> Nobody ever sat down and talked about the problems.

None of the pregnant teenagers had fathers who enforced rules consistently and few (14 percent) reported any parental concern regarding their whereabouts, though the majority (60 percent) felt that their parents were worried about drugs, sex, and "not getting into trouble.'' In contrast, most control women had parents with explicit moral and behavioral goals for their daughters and had among their own future goals social concerns and a close relationship with one's fellow humans. As one control said: ''I want to get a good job so I'll be able to get along in life. As I said before, become a better person and be able to do others some good.'' And another control: ''I want to experiment, to add to my life, taste all the different things around—broaden my perspective.''

None of the pregnant teenagers did. Most of them, by contrast, worried a lot, mostly about money. More than half felt some need for psychotherapy during adolescence, considered it, but did not go. Those who actively looked for help turned more often to professionals (26 percent), while control women sought help from older friends (50 percent).

Very few of the pregnant teenagers (less than one out of four) thought highly of themselves. Though most ''wanted a better life for themselves and their kids,'' they felt that the door to adult life that was opening to their peers had already shut them out. In the words of one young woman, age 18, with one year-old baby and another on the way: ''I always wanted things to be perfect, you know: get married, get my own place, be happy, but nothing seems to be going smoothly. And I feel it is so hard, and now we are going to have two children, and I don't want them to go through what I went through.''

Discussion

While almost all the adolescent delinquents in our study were among the learning disabilities and mental health problems identified by age 10, most of the young women who became pregnant in adolescence showed few if any signs in childhood that they might be prone to have serious interpersonal problems in their teens. This may be due to the limitation of our screening instruments and the perspectives of our informants (mothers and teachers) at age 10. Since the majority of pregnant teenagers in this cohort had negative or at best ambivalent relationships with their parents, especially their mothers, the latter may have been unwilling or unable to communicate a (mutual) lack of understanding between parents and daughters.

There have been only a few other studies of black and white pregnant teenagers on the U.S. mainland which have used unmarried, nonpregnant control women from the same age group, socioeconomic status, and ethnic background to evaluate the contributions of personality factors to adolescent pregnancy (Brunswick 1971; Kane and Lachenbruch 1973). Their findings, like ours with a predominantly Polynesian and Oriental sample, seem to indicate that considerably more emphasis must be placed on dealing with the motivational issues in pregnant adolescents if we are to avoid the high recidivism rate usually associated with adolescent pregnancy. We do not underrate the significance of findings of demographic surveys that have shown that the teenage population most at risk for illegitimate pregnancies comes, for the most part, from the poorest homes with the least educational stimulation—at the rate of 5 percent for white, 9 to 10 percent for nonwhite adolescent women on the mainland (Brunswick 1971; Keeve et al. 1969), and 8 percent in our multiracial sample of women on Kauai.

These demographic factors were among the few signposts we found (as early as age 10), but equally significant was the fact that many of the pregnant teenagers came from a subculture that valued a nurturant maternal role and prized children highly, a characteristic that distinguishes contemporary Hawaiians from other American ethnic groups (Howard et al. 1970).

In May 1971, Hawaii become the first state to allow abortion on request of the woman, but the girls of Hawaiian descent among our pregnant teenagers chose this option least often. Although they constituted nearly half (43 percent) of the teenage pregnancies, part-Hawaiian girls contributed to only 20 percent of the abortions among women of high school age, in contrast to members of other subcultures such as the Japanese (14 percent of teenage pregnancies, 60 percent of abortions) and the Caucasians (R. G. Smith et al. 1971), who chose abortions more frequently. The majority of the pregnant teenagers of Hawaiian descent kept their babies or "hanaied" them to their parents, grandparents, close relatives, or friends—an adoption custom that has persisted in spite of great cultural changes across generations (Howard et al. 1970) and is exemplified by the life story of the young woman in the interview excerpted later in this chapter.

Our data confirm findings by others on white and black teenage mothers (Kane and Lachenbruch 1973) that these are young women for whom pregnancy and motherhood could be a source of gratification and self-esteem but whose ambivalent or negative relationship with parents or parent substitutes and whose sense of powerlessness make pregnancy very stressful.

Of all the groups of youth at risk in this cohort, pregnant teenagers scored in the most external direction on the Novicki Locus of Control Scale. They had little faith that their own actions determined the reinforcement they received. Our findings on rural Kauai are quite similar to the respones of lower-class black and Spanish-speaking teenage mothers and pregnant teenagers in New York's inner city who voiced a lower sense of control over their lives than nonpregnant girls from the same low socioeconomic background (Brunswick 1971).

This feeling of powerlessness that runs through the interview responses of the teenage mothers may well have been an antecedent as well as a correlate of their pregnancy experience. Novicki and Segal (1974) have shown that greater internal control in senior girls in high school is associated with greater perceived affection, security, trust, and physical contact with both father and mother and with greater social involvement with peers—all factors conspicuously missing in the lives of the pregnant teenagers in our study.

If teenage pregnancy and motherhood are steps in the long road to maturity, the provision of options—legalized abortion, adoption, educational programs inside and outside the regular high school programs (home tutoring, evening classes), health care for pregnant women and their infants, family life education, family planning programs—are promising beginnings, but they need to be extended to more of those in need. In this group, few (only about 1 out of 10) received their benefits.

Most of all, educational, health, and social programs need to be bolstered by compassionate attention to the mental health needs of the pregnant teenager to help her overcome her sense of powerlessness—opening doors to life instead of closing them.

Unless she gains a greater sense of control over her own life, the poignant statement by the pregnant teenage mother in this chapter is apt to be repeated, at some future time, by her *own* daughter: "Well, all of my life, nothing goes right." She continued, recalling earlier years: "I wanted to belong to clubs like that a lot, but my parents didn't want me to. I guess they didn't have enough time to take me and bring me home." She left school ("I liked high school") and attended night school while pregnant

with her second baby—"it [night school] was all right"—obtained
a diploma, and now planned to go back to work after the birth of
her second child:

> Before I got married, I was working in a hotel and I was a waitress. I
> was planning to go back and work after my first baby, but then I got
> pregnant again. I told my husband that it's going to be hard for him
> to work and to have to support me and the two kids and himself, so
> it's best that I go back to work. [*Question*] A couple of months after
> the baby's born. His greatgrandmother is willing to take care of
> them, but if I wait until they're much older, it would be hard for
> her . . . maybe when my second baby is about a year old.

Asked about friends:

> I liked to do things with a group of people. But sometimes I would
> just want to be alone and think things over. [*Question*] I had a best
> friend. But then, after I got married, we just drifted apart. [*Question*] Yes, things really sort of change. [*And how well do you think
> you get along with other people*?] Oh, I guess, all right.

The interviewer asks her to tell something about her family:

> Actually, when I was born, my mother wasn't married to my father,
> so I was adopted by my grandparents, my mother's parents. Then
> my mother got married to a guy. We all lived in a three-bedroom
> house, three families living in one house . . . I lived with them till I
> was about ten. Then my mother got married to this other guy and
> she and my brothers and sisters moved to Honolulu . . . and I
> stayed on Kauai, and my stepfather and my cousins and me, we
> moved to another house. And then when I was about twelve, thir-
> teen, fourteen I started to make troubles, running away and not
> even coming home. My stepfather thought I was screwing around
> and wouldn't accept the fact that I was growing up and wouldn't let
> me go out with any of my friends. So I lived with my sister and after
> that I stopped going to school. My sister, she's very strict, but it's
> for the best. She's much more understanding than the others—she'd
> talk to me, explain things. . . . When I was much younger I used to
> have fights with my brothers and sisters, and my real mother would
> feel bad because they were my brothers and sisters and I shouldn't
> do that. But then my grandparents used to spank me, and she would
> feel bad and she would say she shouldn't have put me up for adop-
> tion, and if she didn't, I would be in Honolulu with her right now. I
> don't know, I guess she felt bad. [*Question*] When I was about
> twelve years old, I found out I was adopted. Then I remembered

when I was small, there was this guy that would come over and be with them, and he was my father, and my grandmother would call me in the house and ask me what he was telling me, and I would tell her that he was my father. She'd tell me, "Don't believe he's your father," that my grandfather was my father. But then on my birthdays he would always come over and take me to the store and I could choose anything I wanted. I grew up and I found out he was my father. . . . Then after I got married my godmother told me he was going back to the Philippine Islands. So I tried to find out where he lived and saw him the day before he left and he cried. He didn't really want to go. . . . I wrote to him for a couple of months, and the last time I wrote to him, he didn't answer. I don't know. [*You've had so many parents and parent substitutes. How do you feel about it?*] I feel that all my life I've been moved here and moved there, and I guess I'll never really be able to understand it all. Guess I'll never be able to settle down. Even now. My mother and father-in-law got a divorce, and now we're living with my mother-in-law. We hope to find a place of our own, but it's so hard.

She said that she only wanted to have the two children and "after this I'm going to Family Planning until I'm old enough and then I'll go to a doctor about fixing myself." Questioned about how she felt these experiences had influenced her, she continued:

I guess I was being locked up so much that I wanted to be free, and then I ended up in the same position, and instead of doing what I want to do I'm home with kids and not having my freedom like I wanted. I started my life all over though, you know, bringing up kids and hoping that they don't go through what I went through. [*What do you think you can do to make it different?*] Be more understanding, because my parents, when I wanted to talk to them about a problem, they would just shout "Don't bother!", you know. If my children come to me with a problem, I would try to explain it much better and be easy on them. [*Question*] When I was young I used to ask questions, and they [parents] would just hit me and say I was dumb, acting like a child. . . . Then when I started living with my sister, we'd talk and we had a much better understanding than my parents . . . she helps me a lot. . . . Now, if I do need help, you know, with my in-laws or something, she will always talk to me and comfort me, and tell me to just try and hold on until something much better turns out. [*Asked how her grandparents (stepparents) had gotten across ideas about behavior, values, and so forth.*] They really didn't tell me what is good or bad, they just wanted me to stay home, *not* go here and *not* go there and *not* do this and *not* do that. It was really hard. . . . When I was with them, I was in high school and the only kind of girls I knew were the kind that wanted to meet other girls and fight and things like that. I was in a group of girls like that, although I didn't start fights or anything. I felt that if I hang around girls like that they would protect me all of the time, they took care of girls like that. I was getting worse and worse, and my parents had so many problems, I turned to my sister. . . . When I went with her, she said dress length had to be just right, you know, just above the knee, no smoking, no foul language. It was a big change. . . . She let me go out much more than my parents would, although I would have to be home at a certain time. She had to know where I was, who I was with, and what we were doing. [*Question*] We discussed some rules, especially my brother-in-law. He was the kind and understanding type. Whenever I would have a problem and my sister would be busy running in and out, I would talk to my brother-in-law and he would talk it out with me.

And about punishment:

My sister she is very strong-minded and when you're punished, you're punished. If I would go out and say I will be home at a certain time and I don't, my sister would put the rules down and punish me and not let me go out for a month or so. And if in that month a good friend of mine would ask me to go out and I would say "I was a good girl," she'd just say, "I don't care. You're punished and that's all."

Evaluating herself, she indicated that "emotionally I'm weak." Her goals? "I just want to be a good mother and wife . . . get a better life for myself and my kids." And again: "Well, I guess now I want to straighten out myself and get things right for the kids. I guess the only person who really put things right was my sister, she put things on my mind to straighten me out. . . . I went through a lot and I can admit it—if any girl would come to me I'd help out as much as I could as I don't want them to go through what I did."

CHAPTER 9
The Community Response

This chapter focuses on the steps taken by the educational, health, and social service agencies as well as the judicial system on Kauai to deal with serious learning and behavior problems in adolescence among the youth born in 1955—as they were reported in the agencies' records. We will also take a look at the main sources of support and counsel mentioned by the youth in the 18-year interview—peers, older friends, parents—and examine their judgment of the effectiveness of intervention during adolescence.

In comparison with other communities of similar size and population on the mainland, the island of Kauai has been very fortunate in having a great variety of community agencies and volunteer organizations which concern themselves with the needs of children and youth, which are easily accessible, and which open their doors to all, regardless of race, sex, and socioeconomic status. Neighborly *kokua* ("cooperation") is generously practiced to an extent unknown in many of the big cities of the United States (see Chapter 2).

In our earlier follow-up studies we had found no social class differences in the use of health services by the mothers and children in this cohort (Werner, Bierman, and French 1971). An examination of the agency records also failed to reveal significant social class differences between youth with serious learning and behavior problems who received the benefit of some positive intervention by educational and social service agencies during adolescence and those who did not.

As Table 24 suggests, the efforts of the various community agencies tended to go toward helping those who perceived the least emotional support in their families, who worried the most, and who had the greatest conflict feelings.

Among the youth for whom there was some recorded community agency intervention, a significantly higher proportion (70 percent) were dissatisfied with the education they had received and lacked realistic educational plans beyond high school (73 percent) compared to those who did not receive such intervention. A significantly lower proportion (19 percent) of the treated youth with problems had definite vocational plans and a very high proportion (83 percent) worried about their future.

A very low proportion (10 percent) of the youth who received some intervention by community agencies had mothers who wanted their sons and daughters to define their own goals, and the majority (65 percent) viewed their fathers as nonsupportive. Half came from families where there was a great deal of conflict and had themselves great conflict feelings.

Youth Who Received Help

It had been agreed earlier (in 1966) that the findings of our screening and assessment at age 10, especially those of significance for individual children, should be made available to everyone con-

Table 24   Differences Between Problem Youth with and without Intervention by Community Agencies on Interview at Age 18

Dimension	Treated Youth (%) (N=28)	Untreated Youth (%) (N=101)	Chi Square*	p
Satisfied with education	30	59	5.01	.05
Realistic educational plans beyond high school	27	65	7.03	.01
Definite vocational plans	19	50	5.42	.02
Mother wants child to decide goal	10	40	6.02	.02
Father viewed as nonsupportive	65	37	4.40	.05
Family argues without resolution	50	21	8.64	.01
Worries (much)	83	57	4.25	.05
(Very) great conflict feelings	48	24	4.04	.05
Received psychotherapy	32	8	4.28	.05
Received professional help (M.D., psychiatrist, psychologist)	30	8	10.03	.01

* df = 1.

cerned. Letters with suggestions for follow-up and referrals to special agencies went to the parents of all the children at risk. Reports of the special diagnostic examinations went to the child's physicians and psychological test scores went to the Department of Education. With parental consent, diagnostic reports were sent to specific community agencies, such as the Division of Mental Health of the local Department of Health, if the parents initiated a follow-up contact.

In spite of these efforts, only a third of all the youth at risk received some professional help or psychotherapy, but the incidence of agency intervention varied greatly with the type of problem. It should also be noted that the agencies were not always aware of our previous findings or each other's evaluations and activities.

The largest proportion of those who received assistance came from the group diagnosed as mentally retarded by age 10. More than half (14 out of 25) of the MRs were serviced by one or more of the community agencies during adolescence, predominantly by the Department of Education's Office of Guidance and Special Services and the Department of Social Services and Housing's Division of Vocational Rehabilitation.

The next most frequently served group was youth diagnosed as having learning disabilities at age 10: Slightly less than half (10 out of 22) received some form of professional help during their teen years, predominantly by the Office of Guidance and Special Services, the high school counselors, and a few by the Department of Health.

Less than half (10 out of 25) of the youth considered in need of long-term mental health services at age 10 had the benefit of some form of professional intervention by community agencies during adolescence. Most were assisted by the Office of Guidance and Special Services, only a small proportion by the Division of Mental Health.

By the time of the 18-year follow-up, a third (15 out of 45) of the youth with new problems that arose during adolescence had received some help, either through the Family Court, Mental Health, or Special Services. This was the *only* group among the youth at risk in which proportionately more boys than girls benefited from community intervention. Among the teenage pregnancies only 10 percent took advantage of professional help.

Of all the youth with behavior problems, those who had been considered in need of short-term mental health services at age 10 received the least amount of professional assistance by community agencies. Only one-tenth (6 out of 60) among the SMH cases received some help (from Special Services, Mental Health, and Vocational Rehabilitation).

Lest we put the responsibility for this state of affairs entirely on the community agencies or the parents whose consent was needed for intervention, it must be kept in mind that with the exception of about half the new problems in adolescence, only a minority of those with childhood learning and behavior problems perceived a *need* for professional help during adolescence. About four-fifths (85 percent) of the SMH youth and the majority of the LMH youth (60 percent) and LD youth (69 percent) diagnosed at age 10 stated in the 18-year interview that they had never thought of it. One might also wonder how aware they were of the *availability* of services.

Sources of Help

Tables 25 to 28 summarize the *recorded* action taken by the educational, social services, health, and mental health agencies as well as the judicial system in response to the needs of youth with serious learning and behavior problems in middle childhood and adolescence.

DEPARTMENT OF EDUCATION

Of all the agencies, the Department of Education provided the most direct service to the largest number of adolescents with problems in this cohort. This is a tribute to the efforts of the coordinator of the Office of Guidance and Special Services, the psychological examiners, the speech and hearing specialists, the school social workers, the diagnostic-prescriptive teachers, and the high school counselors, including the Outreach counselors. It also speaks well for the introduction and use of special programs for potential dropouts, including work-motivation classes and special off-campus courses.

As can be seen in Table 25, considerable effort was spent assisting the mentally retarded in the 1955 cohort, 40 percent of whom were helped in adolescence through placement in special classes and learning centers, special therapy, or assignment to counselors.

Table 25   Recorded Action Taken by Department of Education
in Behalf of Youth with Problems (1955 Cohort)

Action	MR (%) (N=25)	LD (%) (N=22)	LMH (%) (N=25)	SMH (%) (N=60)	NP (%) (N=45)
Placement in special class	40.0	4.5	—	—	—
Placement in learning center	8.0	4.5	4.0	2.0	—
Individualized instruction in regular class	—	13.5	8.0	2.0	—
Home tutoring for pregnant females	—	4.0	4.0	—	6.6
Speech therapy	—	9.0	—	—	—
Physical therapy	8.0	—	—	—	—
Assignment to counselor	4.0	18.0	16.0	5.0	4.5
Letter or conference with parents	4.0	13.5	16.0	3.0	—
Detention	4.0	—	4.0	2.0	—
Academic probation	—	4.5	4.0	—	—
Suspension or dismissal from school	—	—	4.0	2.0	—
Referral to other agencies	4.0	4.5	4.0	—	—

Youth with learning disabilities at age 10 were assisted less frequently by the Office of Guidance and Special Services or the counselors during their teen years. About a third (36 percent) received some professional help in the form of counseling, individualized instruction in regular classes, speech therapy, or placement in special classes or learning centers.

Only one out of every five (20 percent) of the youth considered in need of long-term mental health services at age 10 received assistance by the Office of Guidance and Special Services in adolescence. Counseling, conferences with parents, individualized instruction in regular classrooms, or placement in a learning center were the primary means of intervention. Only one out of every ten of the youth considered in need of short-term mental health services at age 10 received the same type of assistance in school during their teen years.

Among the new problems in adolescence, only 10 percent of the pregnant teenagers in this cohort availed themselves of the opportunity to be tutored at home or to attend special evening classes.

POLICE AND FAMILY COURT

Next to the educational system, the judicial system on Kauai was most actively involved in positive intervention among adolescents with behavior problems. Both systems, one might argue, had a

Table 26   Recorded Action Taken by Police and Family Court in Behalf of Youth with Problems (1955 Cohort)

Action	MR (%) (N=25)	LD (%) (N=22)	LMH (%) (N=25)	SMH (%) (N=60)	NP (%) (N=45)
Cited	8.0	4.5	—	3.0	—
Counseled	—	9.0	28.0	3.0	20
Referred to Family Court	16.0	13.5	16.0	8.5	22
Referred to mental health clinic	—	—	8.0	2.0	4.5
Placed in state hospital	—	4.5	—	2.0	4.5
Placed in foster home	8.0	—	8.0	2.0	6.6
Placed on probation	—	9.0	—	—	—
Placed in youth correctional facility	8.0	4.5	4.0	3.0	—
Placed in Job Corps	4.0	4.5	4.0	3.0	—

captive audience and did not have to rely on parental consent and cooperation to the extent necessary for intervention by other community agencies, such as the Divisions of Mental Health and Vocational Rehabilitation. However, the positive steps taken by the police and the Family Court on Kauai are also a tribute to the judge in the Family Court, to the special counselors in the Juvenile Crime Prevention Unit, and to the school relations officer who maintained a liaison between the Police Department and the high schools (see Table 26).

Disproportionately more MRs than any other youth at risk were referred by the police to the Family Court in adolescence and placed under its custody (24 percent seen by the police, 16 percent referred to Family Court). Eight percent of the MRs were subsequently placed in foster homes, 8 percent in the Hawaii Youth Correctional Facility, and 4 percent in the Job Corps.

The Police Department had contact with one out of four (27 percent) among the learning disability cases in adolescence and counseled about 1 out of 10. Half the LDs seen by the police (13.5 percent) were eventually referred to the Family Court. Nine percent of the LDs were placed under the supervision of a probation officer, and 4.5 percent each were placed in the Hawaii State Mental Hospital, the Hawaii Youth Correctional Facility, and the Job Corps respectively.

The Police Department had contact with nearly one-third (32 percent) of the LMH youth during their teen years, counseled 28 percent, and referred 16 percent to the Family Court and 8 percent to the Community Mental Health Clinic. Eight percent of the

LMH youth were subsequently placed in foster homes and 4 percent each in the Hawaii Youth Correctional Facility and the Job Corps.

Youth who were considered in need of short-term mental health services at age 10 had the lowest rate of contacts with the police (17 percent) during adolescence. About 1 out of every 10 was counseled by the police or the Family Court. Subsequently, 3 percent each of the SMH youth were placed in the Hawaii Youth Correctional Facility and the Job Corps, respectively, and 2 percent each were referred to the Kauai Community Mental Health Clinic and the Hawaii State Mental Hospital.

Of all the groups of youth at risk, the new problems in adolescence had the most frequent contacts with the police. One out of every five (20 percent) was counseled by the police; one out of every five (22 percent) was referred to the Family Court. Seven percent were subsequently placed in foster homes and 4.5 percent each were referred to the Kauai Community Mental Health Clinic and the Hawaii State Mental Hospital.

DEPARTMENT OF SOCIAL SERVICES AND HOUSING

As can be seen in Table 27, about half the mentally retarded (44 percent) and approximately one out of every five youth among the other groups at risk (LD=22 percent; LMH=20 percent; SMH=17 percent; NP=17 percent) received some financial assistance by the Department of Social Services and Housing during their teen

Table 27   Recorded Action Taken by Department of Social Services and Housing in Behalf of Youth with Problems (1955 Cohort)

Action	MR (%) (N=25)	LD (%) (N=22)	LMH (%) (N=25)	SMH (%) (N=60)	NP (%) (N=45)
Division of Public Welfare					
Financial assistance	44.0	22	20.0	17.0	17.0
Foster home placement	12.0	—	24.0	7.0	6.6
Referral to other agencies	8.0	—	8.0	3.0	—
Division of Vocational Rehabilitation					
Placed in work-study program	20.0	4.5	4.0	—	2.0
Placed in Job Corps	—	—	—	3.0	—
Placed in Rehabilitation Unlimited Kauai	4.0	—	—	2.0	—
Referral to other agencies	4.0	4.5	4.0	—	—

years, either aid for dependent children or assistance to cover medical costs.

Most of the other intervention efforts in adolescence by the Divisions of Public Welfare and Vocational Rehabilitation centered on youth considered in need of long-term mental health services at age 10 and on the mentally retarded.

The Division of Public Welfare had regular contacts with about one-third of all the LMH youth during their teen years and placed one out of four in foster homes. By comparison, only 12 percent of those in need of short-term mental health services at age 10 and 15 percent of the new problems in adolescence had some form of professional help from the Division of Public Welfare, and only 7 percent in each group were placed in foster homes during adolescence.

The Division of Vocational Rehabilitation did a very effective job of educational and vocational rehabilitation for one out of every four of the mentally retarded in adolescence through placement in work-study programs, the Job Corps, or the sheltered workshop run by a volunteer organization, Rehabilitation Unlimited Kauai. By comparison, less than 5 percent among the other groups of youth at risk (LD, LMH, SMH, NP) were placed in work-study, Job Corps, or other vocational rehabilitation programs during their teen years.

DEPARTMENT OF HEALTH

The Division of Public Health Nursing gave professional assistance to more than half (52 percent) of the mentally retarded in the 1955 cohort during adolescence. Services consisted either in continuation of regular care begun in early childhood or correction of a physical handicap through surgery, braces, wheelchairs, hearing aids, or medication. The division saw one out of every five of the youth diagnosed as having learning disabilities at age 10 in their teens, but only for diagnostic workups which confirmed the presence of organic (central nervous system) damage. These youth were then referred to other agencies.

Few of the mental health problems—12 percent of those considered in need of long-term mental health services and 7 percent of those with short-term mental health needs—were seen by the division in adolescence, mostly to correct minor physical handicaps or for referral to other agencies (see Table 28).

Table 28   Recorded Action Taken by Department of Health in Behalf of Youth with Problems (1955 Cohort)

Action	MR (%) (N=25)	LD (%) (N=22)	LMH (%) (N=25)	SMH (%) (N=60)	NP (%) (N=45)
Division of Mental Health					
Diagnostic workup only	—	9.0	20.0	3.0	—
Individual or Group psychotherapy	—	9.0	8.0	—	4.5
Drug therapy	—	4.5	4.0	—	4.5
Referral to mental hospital or other agencies	—	9.0	12.0	2.0	4.5
Big Sister affiliation	—	5.0	4.0	2.0	10.0
Division of Public Health Nursing					
Condition corrected	8.0	—	8.0	2.0	—
Continuation of regular care	12.0	—	—	—	—
Referral to other agencies	28.0	18.0	4.0	2.0	—

By the time of our 18-year follow-up, the staff of the Division of Mental Health had grown to include two psychiatrists, one clinical psychologist, two social workers, and two paramedical assistants, all with a strong commitment to community mental health, crisis intervention, and the systems approach. Nevertheless, they could reach only 28 percent of the LMH youth and 5 percent of the SMH youth during their teen years. This proportion is *identical* with the one reported in the Robins study of deviant children (1966: 210). Half a century ago, in the early 1920s, 28 percent of all referrals to a municipal child guidance clinic from a lower-class and lower-middle-class white population in St. Louis actually received treatment.

As can be seen from Table 28, about one out of every five of the long-term mental health problems diagnosed in childhood was seen for a diagnostic workup in adolescence. Twelve percent were referred to local hospitals, and 8 percent each were seen at the Community Mental Health Clinic either for individual or group therapy; 4.5 percent of the LMH cases received some form of drug therapy during adolescence.

Few of the few youth (5 percent) in need of short-term mental health services seen by the Division of Mental Health during adolescence received any treatment: 3 percent were seen for diagnostic workups only and 2 percent were referred to the local inpatient program of the Mental Health Service (Mahelona Hospital).

Of the learning disability cases diagnosed at age 10, 13.5 percent were seen by the Community Mental Health Clinic during adolescence—9 percent for diagnostic workups, 9 percent for individual or group therapy, and 4.5 percent for drug therapy.

Four percent each of the new problem cases in adolescence were likewise seen in the Community Mental Health Clinic for individual or group psychotherapy or drug therapy. Four percent were referred to the Hawaii State Mental Hospital.

VOLUNTEER PROGRAMS

Two of the volunteer programs in the community assisted a number of youth with problems in the 1955 cohort during adolescence. One was Rehabilitation Unlimited Kauai, which worked closely with the Division of Vocational Rehabilitation in placing 4 percent of the mentally retarded and 2 percent of the short-term mental health problems in vocational rehabilitation programs and sheltered workshops. The other volunteer programs, Big Sisters and Big Brothers, newly founded in Kauai during the time this cohort came of age, worked closely with the various community agencies. One out of ten among the new problems in adolescence had the benefit of an association with a Big Sister, as did 5 percent of the learning disabilities, 4 percent of the youth diagnosed in need of long-term mental health services at age 10, and 2 percent of those in need of short-term mental health services. Both volunteer groups are examples of promising links between professionals and paraprofessionals in the various community agencies and concerned people of goodwill on the island.

PEERS, PARENTS, AND OLDER FRIENDS

As can be seen from Table 29 peer friends ranked first as a source of help among *all* the groups of youth at risk (as they did among the corresponding control groups without problems). There were, however, some significant differences in the proportion of problem youth who stated in the 18-year interview that they turned to peers for counsel. Two-thirds (67 percent) of those considered in need of long-term mental health services turned to peers for help, in contrast to only about a third (36 percent) of the youth in need of short-term mental health services ($p < .10$) and a third (32 percent) among the new problem cases in adolescence. A smaller proportion of youth with learning disabilities turned to peers than other groups of youth at risk (28 percent). This probably was another indicator of their relative social isolation.

Roughly one-fourth of the children with learning disabilities and mental health problems stated that they turned to their parents for support and counsel, but the proportion was lower (16 percent) among the new problems in adolescence, many of whom had persistent conflicts with parents, parent surrogates, or other authority figures.

Approximately one out of every five youths who had been diagnosed as having learning disabilities or mental health problems at age 10 turned to older friends for counsel during their teen years, but the new problems in adolescence relied on this source of help least frequently.

Among the learning and behavior problems diagnosed in childhood, it was found that professionals, whether teachers, counselors, ministers, psychiatrists, psychologists, or social workers, ranked far below peers, parents, and older friends as sources of help to whom they would spontaneously turn. This trend was reversed among the new problems in adolescence: about one-third had been seen by professionals for help and about one-fourth considered counselors a source of constructive help. This may well reflect a greater awareness of availability of professional help among the youth whose problem arose in adolescence and a greater freedom to turn to these sources, since these youth were not so dependent on parental consent or cooperation as those with learning and behavior problems diagnosed in childhood.

Effectiveness of Intervention

Regarding their judgment of the effectiveness of help given them, overall there were no significant differences between youth with serious behavior and learning problems who had received profes-

Table 29 Sources of Help Reported by Youth with Problems (1955 Cohort)

Source	LD (%) (N=22)	LMH (%) (N=25)	SMH (%) (N=60)	NP (%) (N=45)
Peer friends	28	67	36	32
Parents	28	28	23	16
Older friends	22	22	21	14
Counselors	11	11	18	24
Teachers	17	6	7	—
Ministers	6	—	7	—
Other professionals	—	6	2	32

sional assistance by community agencies during adolescence and problem youth who had to rely only on counsel of peers and parents.

There were, however, differences in the perceived effectiveness of help given in adolescence among the different subgroups of youth at risk. Of all the groups, those with long-term mental health problems contained the highest proportion who felt that emotional support and counsel given them during adolescence helped a lot and made them feel much better (53 percent); nearly half the short-term mental health problems and the new problems interviewed felt the same way.

In contrast, only one out of every five learning disability cases interviewed felt that assistance had helped a lot. Nearly two-thirds stated that it helped only a little. For some 3 to 7 percent among the problem youth it was considered a waste of time.

Risk-Taking or Runaround?

During the decade that the community mental health approach was ushered in (since 1963), much has been made in public statements of the need for cooperation among different helping agencies (Roen 1971). In theory, if not always in practice, all the community agencies on Kauai have long been strongly committed to the interdisciplinary approach of solving problems for and with those who need or seek help.

These are more opportunities for informal exchange of information among concerned professionals on this island than in larger communities. The location of the primary agencies around one square in the county seat, Lihue, is such that a few steps to the next wing or next floor of the same building or across the street will suffice to obtain diagnostic information and decisions on joint intervention that would take weeks and months to achieve in an inner city. Ancillary helping organizations such as Rehabilitation Unlimited Kauai and Big Sisters and Big Brothers are only a few blocks or, at most, a few miles away.

Working in such a setting were dedicated people willing to cut across professional boundaries, to communicate with one another, to trust the judgment of those with skills and experiences different from their own. They were not immobilized by red tape—in short, they took risks.

Alas, we cannot overlook the other side of the coin—the lack of professional cooperation, the inter- and intra-agency jealousies and disagreements which were often at the client's expense. These unfortunately are not documented in our records and can only be speculated on or inferred by the blank spaces and sudden halts to action. From time to time we had to ask ourselves, "What *did* happen here?" The answer might well be found in the statement of one of the young people quoted earlier: "I got the runaround."

In the next chapter we examine how community intervention, parental support, and the efforts and communication skills of the youth at risk contributed to changes in status. We then discuss the implications of our findings for the delivery of services to children and youth with serious learning and behavior problems. This discussion appears to be timely in light of the mass screening and assessment of children at developmental risk mandated by the 1970 Developmental Disabilities Act and by the 1967 Amendment to Title XIX of the Social Security Act, which aims at early and periodic screening, diagnosis, and treatment of all eligible Medicaid individuals under the age of 21.

CHAPTER 10
Changes in Status

Two psychologists read independently the case histories and descriptions of the child's behavior that had led to the recommendations for long- or short-term mental health services or placement in learning disability classes at age 10 for the purpose of assessing change in status. They compared each case history with the agency records during adolescence and interview ratings made of the same youth at age 18, with special attention to ratings of self-esteem, degree of self-insight, absence or presence of conflict, the quality of social and family life, and the realism of educational and vocational plans. A few cases, who could not be reached for the interview because they refused to cooperate or had moved beyond our reach to the mainland (about 10 percent), were rated on the basis of their agency records—if these records were reasonably complete.

In 90 out of the original 102 youth at risk at age 10 (88 percent), the psychologists were able to make an independent judgment on change in status, i.e., whether there appeared to be evidence for improvement or whether the problem had continued or worsened. Overall agreement on these ratings was very satisfactory (91 percent). In the few cases (8 out of 90) in which there was some disagreement, both psychologists considered the 10-year and 18-year evidence together and arrived at a joint judgment.

Rate of Improvement

LD YOUTH

Among the youth considered in need of placement in learning disability classes at age 10, only one out of four was judged improved by age 18. The improvement rate was slightly (but not significantly) higher for those LD cases who had some help by community agencies: One out of three in this group was rated improved. There were no social class differences between those whose status had remained unchanged or deteriorated and those who had improved, but significantly more males than females ($p < .03$) were among the improved LD cases. None of the girls in this group had improved in status from age 10 to age 18, in contrast to 40 percent of the boys.

LMH YOUTH

One out of three youth considered in need of long-term mental health services at age 10 was judged improved by age 18. The improvement rate was higher (but not significantly so) among those who had some assistance by community agencies: One out of two in this group was rated improved. There were no sex or socioeconomic differences between those whose status had remained unchanged or deteriorated and those who had improved in the span between 10 and 18 years.

SMH YOUTH

The improvement rate for the SMH group, which had been exposed to the least amount of intervention by community agencies, was the highest among all the groups of youth at risk. Even among the untreated, 6 out of 10 improved during adolescence. There were no sex differences between those in need of short-term mental health services at age 10 who had improved and those whose status had remained unchanged or deteriorated, but there was a tendency ($p < .07$) for proportionately more middle-class than lower-class youth among the SMH cases to improve in the period between 10 and 18. Seventy-seven percent of the middle-class youth, but only 50 percent of the poor, were judged improved during their teen years.

Family and Interpersonal Variables

In Tables 30 to 32 we present a summary of significant differences between improved and unimproved cases in each group that emerged from the 18-year interview. Most of the responses deal with the youths' perception of the family climate and of the support and understanding received from parents and peers, as well as their assessment of their strong and weak points.

IMPROVED VS. UNIMPROVED LD CASES

More unimproved than improved LD cases described their mothers in negative terms and reported that their parents had little or no influence on them. Significantly more of the improved LD cases found their mothers easy to talk to and viewed them as supportive of their ideas and plans, treating their offspring as separate individuals worthy of respect. In contrast, most of the unimproved cases viewed both their mothers and their fathers as nonsupportive. More of the improved LD cases reported that structure and rules were of importance in their family and that both their mothers and their fathers were consistent in enforcing these rules.

More improved LD cases described themselves as doing well in school and considered hard work and perseverance as their strong points. In contrast, significantly more of the unimproved LD cases regarded not being a good student their weak point and reported that they had not done as well as they should while in high school (see Table 30).

Case C. Y.: This youth, an improved LD case, reflects some of these points. We found many of the LD cases to be relatively nonverbal in interview, but the message was clear. Speaking of high school he said: "I like high school, it's good . . . and I'm not doing that bad, no more F's on report cards. I'm satisfied. It is important for the future to do well. I plan to be a mechanic . . . take a two-year course at Kauai Community College. [*Question*] Our family? We go on outings, visit the family, go to the beach together on weekends. . . . My mom, she's good, she's real kind. [*Question*] Father? Same. . . . I think I'm like my parents in certain things I do, more like my father." He replied "good" when asked how they got along, and indicated that he felt "real close" to them. "They understand me plenty." Parents were reported to have emphasized "education," but "they leave it up to me what I want to be. . . . We have to do duties at

Table 30 Differences Between Improved (*N*=4) and Unimproved (*N*=16) LD Cases on 18-Year Interview

Interview Response*	Fisher's Exact Probability Test†
More I than U doing (very) well in school.	.01
More U than I not doing well as they should.	.03
More U than I report father had little or no influence on them.	.04
More I than U report structure very important in family.	.02
More I than U report father consistent in enforcing rules (most of the time).	.02
More I than U report mother consistent in enforcing rules (most or all of the time).	.02
More U than I view father as nonsupportive.	.05
More U than I view mother as nonsupportive.	.04
More I than U view mother as supportive of most plans.	.003
More I than U view "hard work, perseverance" as strong point.	.02
More U than I view being "not a good student" as weak point.	.01

* I=improved; U=unimproved.
† df=1.

home, chores, take turns on them all. . . . My mother says this is the way it's going to be [chores], and we get punishment if we don't do it. [*Question*] Lower allowance . . . we don't argue that much. . . . If we start to quarrel, we try to straighten everything out. [*Question*] Talk about it. . . . My strong points? Mostly I do a job well, work good [*conscientious*]. . . . My weak point? Having trouble staying in school before, with my grades."

Case H. J.: In contrast this youth, not improved, says: "First I liked high school, but my mind wasn't made up if I wanted to go to school. I stopped as a sophomore, signed up for Job Corps but didn't go, came back to high school and didn't like it. I had pretty bad grades, F was lowest and C highest. It [school] was important, but I just didn't care." About parental behavior and concerns: "Oh, my mother. She's something else—she gets kind of moody every other day. . . . My father, he's real quiet, likes to sleep though. . . . I don't feel I'm that close to my mother, nor my father . . . sometimes they understand me, sometimes they don't . . . we grumble all the time. I guess my mother has influenced me the most, but she goes after me all the time for everything, says things and I don't even know them. My father doesn't bother at all."

"I don't know what they want me to be. . . . We have to do chores. Mother tells us and we agree on which. But we don't follow the rules sometimes, then nothing is done and another hassle begins again. [*Question*] Oh, boy, it's really something then . . . everyone gets mad . . . they don't sit down and work it out, we go our own way . . . and that's where the whole trouble comes from." And later: "I worry about what's going to become of me, I sure do worry much. . . . I got help once from a teacher, but after that I never thought about it any other time. After that I thought I had to help myself, instead of depending on other people to help."

IMPROVED VS. UNIMPROVED LMH CASES

More improved than unchanged youth in the LMH group were frank in discussing their father and mother, described *both* parents in positive tones, and showed a preference for modeling themselves after them. Significantly more improved LMH youth reported that their mothers and fathers were easy to talk to and that *both* parents had influenced them much.

> **Case O. R.:** This male LMH case, improved, had the following comments about his parents: "My mother, she is real good, real friendly. . . . My father's just about the same, he's really generous, anything you want he gives you. We get along real well and are real close. . . . I guess I'm more like my mother as a person. If I say something, I really mean it, just like her. I don't go back on my word. But I really like the way my father is generous, I follow up on that. If someone likes something I get, I give without grumbling or anything . . . they understand pretty good . . . maybe there's a small generation gap because of my long hair, but not much . . . we talk things over quite often." Questioned about family rules and discipline, he felt things had been "about average." "They showed me what to do and they taught me right and wrong by punishment. . . . Sometimes I come home late at night, 'OK, you stay home next day.' I don't mind, it was my fault. But there isn't much punishment."

While the families of most of the unimproved LMH youth talked little together and parents set rules without consulting their offspring, the improved LMH cases reported a different family climate: Their families discussed disagreements and arrived at solutions acceptable to all. Moral precepts were taught by parental example and consistent enforcement of rules.

There was a significant difference between improved and unchanged LMH youth in their perception of parental support and understanding: More improved cases stated that both their father and their mother tried to understand them as separate individuals and were supportive of them. The unimproved LMH cases reported the contrary: Most in this group had parents with low expectations for their offspring and mothers who left it up to their children to decide what they wanted to do with their futures. This seems to have had an effect on the youths' educational plans: Most of the improved LMH cases looked forward to some education beyond high school, including college; most of the unchanged LMH youth did not.

Significantly more of the unimproved LMH cases reported that their fathers had personal problems and that they had negative relationships with their siblings. They also had fewer peer friends than LMH youth whose status improved between ages 10 and 18 (see Table 31). As one of them said:

> Me and him [father] don't get along that good. I mean I can't look up to him because he's always razing me down. He told me, "The door is open, you can go." . . . Once I did. It's worse when he drinks . . . bad feelings come out. I'll try to do it differently with my kids. . . . I don't get along too well with my brothers and sisters. There are twelve children and I am the thirteenth. But I'm the oldest. I hate bullies, but I think I'm one bully to them.

IMPROVED VS. UNIMPROVED SMH CASES

Youth considered in need of short-term mental health services at age 10 had the highest rate of improvement during adolescence, even without any professional intervention. Among all the groups of youth at risk, the improved SMH cases were differentiated from the unimproved by the largest number of interview responses (see Table 32).

The perceptions of the improved SMH cases regarding their parents and the general family climate were similar to those of the improved LD and LMH cases: They were frank and responsive in discussing both their father and their mother, perceived their parents in a positive way, and liked to model themselves after them.

While most of the unimproved SMH youth saw little or no

Table 31   Differences Between Improved (*N*=6) and Unimproved (*N*=14) LMH Cases on 18-Year Interview

Interview Response*	Fisher's Exact Probability Test†
More I than U plan to go to college.	.02
More I than U would like father as model.	.01
More I than U describe father in positive tones.	.003
More I than U describe mother in positive tones.	.02
More I than U report father easy to talk to.	.02
More I than U report mother easy to talk to.	.02
More I than U report mother has occupational goals for S.	.02
More I than U report father has influenced them much.	.01
More I than U report mother has influenced them much.	.03
More I than U report family discusses disagreements and arrives at acceptable resolution.	.03
More U than I report family talks little together.	.01
More I than U report father expects some training beyond high school for child, including college.	.05
More U than I report mother leaves it up to child.	.05
More I than U report father understands them.	.02
More I than U report mother understands them.	.01
More I than U view father as supportive.	.001
More I than U view mother as supportive.	.003
More I than U frank in discussing father.	.05
More I than U report fathers have no problems.	.05
More U than I report negative relation with siblings.	.03

* I=improved; U=unimproved.
† df=1.

Table 32   Differences Between Improved (*N*=25) and Unimproved (*N*=16) SMH Cases on 18-Year Interview

Interview Response*	Chi Square	df	*p*
More U than I want only high school graduation or less.	7.81	1	.01
More I than U want college	13.84	1	.01
More I than U satisfied with educational achievement.	6.96	2	.05
More I than U want to be like father or have his attributes.		1	.02†
More I than U want to be like mother or have her attributes.		1	.02†
More I than U see father as (mainly) positive.	5.80	1	.02
More I than U report father easy to talk to most or all of the time.	6.79	1	.01
More I than U report mother easy to talk to most or all of the time.	14.51	1	.01
More U than I report no similarity to father.		1	.01†
More U than I report no similarity to mother.		1	.01†

Table 32   (Continued)

Interview Response*	Chi Square	df	p
More I than U report mother has influenced them (very) much.	19.25	1	.01
More I than U report families discuss disagreements and arrive at solution acceptable to all.	9.42	1	.01
More U than I report families talk little together.	10.60	1	.01
More I than U report families talk much together.	6.79	1	.01
More I than U report parents talk over moral issues and encourage child's own thinking.	6.89	1	.01
More I than U report parents set rules by consulting children.		1	.01†
More I than U have father who supports educational goals that include college.		1	.004†
More I than U have mother who supports educational plans that include college.		1	.004†
More I than U have father who listens and treats S as individual; more U than I have father uninterested in son.		1	.008†
More I than U have mother who listens, tries to understand, treats son as individual; more U than I have mother unconcerned, doesn't understand.		1	.008†
More I than U have father who supports child in most things; more U than I have father who disagrees or is opposed.		1	.01†
More I than U have mother who supports son in most things; more U than I have mother who is uninterested, disagrees, or opposes child's plans.		1	.001†
More I than U report equal involvement in family and friends.	8.20	1	.01
More I than U frank and responsive in discussing father.	15.19	1	.01
More I than U frank and responsive in discussing mother.	15.19	1	.01
More I than U turn to peers for help.		1	.05†
More I than U turn to parents for help.		1	.02†
More I than U felt they were helped a lot.		1	.01†

* I=improved; U=unimproved.
† Fisher's exact probability test.

similarity between themselves and their fathers and mothers, significantly more of the improved SMH cases reported that their fathers and mothers had influenced them a great deal. They had found their parents to be good listeners and easy to talk to and felt that they had tried to understand them. Most of the improved youth perceived both their father and their mother as supportive; most of the unimproved SMH cases felt that their father and mother were unconcerned about them or opposed them. More of the improved than the unchanged SMH youth considered their parents a major source of help when they had problems, and they valued the parental assistance given to them.

Significantly more of the improved SMH youth reported that their families discussed things together, including disagreements that were settled in a way acceptable to all: Their parents talked over moral issues with them and encouraged their children's own opinions; rules were arrived at by consultation with the children.

More of the improved than the unchanged SMH cases reported an equal involvement in family and friends. Peer friends were a major source of help when they needed advice for a problem.

Most of the improved SMH cases were satisfied with their educational achievement and planned to go on to college, in line with the expectations of *both* parents, who supported educational goals beyond high school graduation. In contrast, a high proportion of the unchanged SMH youth appeared satisfied with high school education or even less.

Last, but not least, more of the improved than unchanged SMH youth considered hard work and perseverance as their main asset. This strong point was mentioned more often among *all* the youth at risk whose status had improved between the ages of 10 and 18, regardless of the extent of their educational and mental health needs at age 10.

> **Case R. B.:** This SMH youth portrays many of the characteristics and comments noted in our improved cases. Originally considered in need of short-term mental health services at age 10, with complaints of anxiety, tenseness, and academic underachievement, he was the second of six children raised in a family rated very high in emotional support by our 10-year-study staff. Interviewed at age 18, he reported an active high school career with many extracurricular activities as well as a part-time job. He felt high school was "good, but I'm glad I have to go through it only once—pressure can be heavy. I didn't get what I really wanted out of it and think I could have done better if I really buckled down [grades were average: C's and a few B's]. I could have been on the Honor Roll." Future plans included a four-year college, although he expressed some anxiety, stating he was "sort of afraid to go to college in Honolulu as it's too big."

Residuals of his earlier symptoms showed through also in his comments about his worries: "Most of all I worry how I do in school and when we have family problems and stuff I worry about how we can work it out financially." He indicated that he got help "most of the time from my parents— that's about all. I don't like to go out and make my problems that evident and make it known here and there. It helps to talk with parents. They like to help me out any way they can, and I like telling someone what's bothering me. . . . I talked to counselors in high school when I was deciding about college, thought they could help more than parents, but only about school."

Describing his parents he said: "My mother, well, she's understanding—a warm affectionate person. . . . My father? Well, he's the head of the house. He listens to us and tries to help us out with problems. I find he's very understanding. I feel close enough that I can go up and talk to him and tell him of problems and ask for advice. I think I'm more like my father, but I'm closer to my mother. I'm very close to her." He said that his parents had stressed "work, study hard in school so I could make something of myself—it's a backbreaking world, so get a good education, get a good job and support your family . . . but whatever you want to do is fine with us. . . . They didn't stress any particular job, just make something of yourself. We had rules in our family . . . each of us had a job to do . . . father mostly made them and was pretty consistent about it, mostly it's cutting our wings when we don't do it, my brother is grounded now. . . . We do have arguments, usually get loud and that's all. We try to settle on some kind of agreement, each tries to prove his point . . . we resolve it by getting the facts out . . . we try to settle it, not let it go. . . . Our family is very open about most things." In addition to his parents he expressed positive feelings toward siblings with particular feeling of closeness to his older brother: "He's helped me out in schoolwork and like when I get in fights, talks to me and helps out."

Evaluating himself, he indicated his strong points: "Well, I find when I want something and want it bad enough, I can get it . . . no one can stop me." And his weak points: "I know my weak points are sometimes I can be too overbearing . . . really make a pest of myself. . . . I recognize this and try to control it. . . . I'm a very open-minded sort of a person, can listen to people's problems and see both sides of it, see how and why they feel as they do. If something really gets me going, I can lose my head fast but other than that I can stay pretty cool. In terms of my personality I feel I have a good one—at times I can be overbearing, but I find I can control that and be a better person." He had incorporated parental goals: "The main thing is to get myself settled in a good job first. I want to get a good education for one thing and settle down someday and get married and have a couple of children . . . and when I'm financially well off, travel. I want to see this world before I leave it. I want to see as much as I can."

In contrast is the following case:

Case B. R.: This unimproved male at age 10 was "very shy, lacking in self-confidence, feelings easily hurt" and still bedwetting several times a week. He was the fifth of eight children in a family rated low in emotional support at that time. Reviewing his own family relationships, he said that he did not think he was like either parent and did not think he wanted to be. Describing his mother, he commented: "I cannot tell. She is nice, but if you make her mad, it's something different. She's got a temper. [*Father?*] He don't bother. He just keeps away out of trouble. I hardly see my parents. I hardly stay around. I come and they're sleeping, except Sunday, but I go out and just say 'hi' 'and g'bye.' I never see my father hardly, only about two or three days. I never did talk to him. . . . Most of the time my mother and I are close. She's always concerned about my health, my asthma." His family just "tells me to keep out of trouble." He recalled no rules. Regarding family disagreements: "We grumble, just cool down after a while, go out of the house, drive the car away, come back and it's all over . . . we don't talk."

He felt his parents had left what he wanted to be "up to me," but his plans were indefinite. He thought he "might go to Kauai Community College next year and take up body and fender mechanics, but was not really satisfied with high school. "I cannot learn this way. I think I have to go out and learn myself . . . maybe someday I might learn something I really like." His goals included "keeping out of trouble," "being happy," and "marriage when I reach the age and when it's time." He expressed considerable concern about his asthma—"I cannot explain how I get it. I am ashamed to even go to the doctor. I feel ashamed as I'm sick and it's not nice and I can't stop wheezing."

His only source of help had been his girlfriend—"I always talk to her and it helps." Questioned about whether he'd ever felt the need for additional help, he told the interviewer: "I never thought of it. You see, I never did talk to nobody except you for the first time. To tell the truth maybe I should, but I'm ashamed."

Table 33 summarizes the interview responses that differentiated significantly between the improved and unchanged problem cases when we combined all diagnostic categories (LD, LMH, SMH).

A father with many personal problems was more common among the unimproved learning and behavior problems than among those who improved between ages 10 and 18. This threw a shadow across the whole family: There was little talk or parental support and understanding, little concern about the offspring's fate, and little consistent enforcement of rules. The impact of the family climate was also felt in the future aspirations and worries of the youth themselves: Significantly more of the improved looked forward to a "happy marriage" of their own or, in the case of the girls, a combination of career and marriage.

In contrast, most of the unimproved youth had vague worries about their future. Significantly more in this group reported that they went occasionally or regularly for therapy, but professional intervention was not in their judgment effective. More of the unimproved felt that the assistance given them helped only a little (or not at all); significantly more of the improved youth reported that the counsel of peers, parents, or professionals had helped a lot and made them feel much better.

Improved Vs. Unimproved Youth on Group Tests

In Table 34 we present a summary of mean scores on the SCAT, STEP, CPI, and Novicki Locus of Control Scale which differentiated significantly between youth with serious learning and behavior problems who had improved by age 18 and those who had not. Differences between the improved and the unimproved youth on the CPI were confirmed by both *t* tests and discriminant function analysis.

Youth who improved during adolescence had generally better communication skills than those whose status did not change. Mean scores on the verbal scale of the SCAT and the reading and writing scales of the STEP were significantly higher for the improved than the unimproved youth when all three diagnostic categories (LD, LMH, SMH) were combined. The difference in verbal communication skills was especially pronounced between those with short-term mental problems at age 10 who improved without any intervention during adolescence and those SMH cases who did not.

Youth with serious learning and behavior problems whose status had improved in adolescence also scored significantly higher than the unimproved learning and behavior problems on three CPI scales: sociability, responsibility, and achievement via conformance. High scorers on these three dimensions are described as being more planful, responsible, dependable, resourceful, and efficient; as more outgoing and enterprising; as valuing cooperation, persistence, and intellectual activity and achievement. Low scorers on these three scales are characterized as being more submissive and passive; as more immature, undercontrolled, and impulsive; as more insecure and opinionated; and as easily disorganized under stress.

There was also a significant difference between improved and unchanged learning disability cases on the CPI scales of communality and intellectual efficiency. The LD cases who improved

Table 33   Differences Between Improved (*N*=35) and Unimproved (*N*=46) Youth at Risk (LD, LMH, SMH combined) on 18-Year Interview

Interview Response*	Chi Square	df	*p*
More I than U plan to go to college.	28.35	1	.01
More I than U want interesting work.	4.05	1	.05
More U than I dissatisfied with education received.	5.96	2	.05
More I than U proud of educational achievement.	10.53	2	.01
More U than I intimate only with same sex.	3.93	1	.05
More I than U want to model after father or have his attributes.	9.54	1	.01
More I than U want to model after mother or have her attributes.	5.99	1	.02

Table 33   (Continued)

Interview Response*	Chi Square	df	p
More I than U see father in positive way.	13.48	1	.01
More I than U see mother in positive way.	9.90	1	.01
More I than U report father easy to talk to.	28.71	1	.01
More I than U report mother easy to talk to.	22.34	1	.01
More U than I say mother has no specific goals for them.	5.71	1	.02
More I than U report father influenced them much.	22.46	2	.01
More I than U report mother influenced them much.	33.54	2	.01
More I than U report family handles disagreements through discussion and compromise.	16.20	1	.01
More U than I report family argues without resolution.	5.75	1	.02
More I than U report family talks together considerably.	17.23	2	.01
More I than U report parents transmit ethics: By example.	5.36	1	.05
By discussion of moral issues and encouraging child's own thinking.	8.54	1	.01
More I than U report rules of great importance in family.	6.67	1	.01
More U than I report parents set rules without consulting child.	7.74	1	.01
More I than U report father consistently enforces rules most or all of the time.	6.02	1	.02
More I than U report mother consistently enforces rules most or all of the time.	7.02	1	.02
More I than U report father expects college attendance for child.	4.17	1	.05
More U than I satisfied with high school.	5.95	1	.02
More I than U report mother expects college attendance from child.	4.85	1	.05
More U than I have mother satisfied with high school education for child.	8.65	1	.01
More U than I have mother who leaves goals up to child.	5.84	1	.02
More I than U report father understands them; more U than I view father as uninterested.	10.52	1	.01
More I than U report mothers understand them; more U than I view mother as uninterested.	16.35	1	.01
More I than U view father as supportive; more U than I view father as nonsupportive.	25.39	2	.01
More I than U view mother as supportive; more U than I view mother as nonsupportive.	41.60	2	.01
More I than U have equal involvement in family and friends.	11.21	1	.01
More U than I have difficulty being frank about father.	20.09	1	.01
More U than I have difficulty being frank about mother.	18.17	1	.01
More I than U report father had no problems.	4.80	1	.05
More I than U have "happy marriage" as future goal.	5.28	1	.02
More U than I have vague worries about future.	4.02	1	.05

* I=improved; U=unimproved.

Table 34   Differences Between Improved (*N*=35) and Unimproved (*N*=29) Youth at Risk on Measures of Interpersonal Competency, Ability, and Achievement at Grade 12

Scale	Improved		Unimproved		t	p
	Mean	SD	Mean	SD		
LD Cases						
CPI communality	20.88	4.67	15.33	1.97	3.02	.01
LMH Cases						
CPI achievement via conformance	19.57	4.24	14.50	4.37	2.12	.05
SMH Cases						
CPI responsibility	22.09	4.15	19.08	2.36	2.74	.01
Locus of control	12.35	3.99	15.08	4.80	1.77	.08
SCAT verbal	35.47	26.63	15.50	10.63	3.04	.005
SCAT quantitative	42.00	29.00	23.58	22.26	2.04	.05
SCAT total	37.67	27.64	16.33	15.17	2.86	.007
STEP reading	40.33	29.28	16.23	18.32	2.95	.006
STEP writing	43.14	25.96	19.69	19.07	3.06	.005
LD, LMH, SMH combined						
CPI responsibility	21.14	4.32	19.07	3.29	2.14	.03
SCAT verbal	34.97	28.68	23.56	14.01	2.30	.03
STEP reading	33.61	28.30	16.53	15.78	2.92	.005
STEP writing	36.13	26.62	17.15	15.83	3.37	.001

during adolescence had learned to use their intellectual resources better and their judgment more efficiently than those whose problems persisted, though there was no difference between the two groups in mean intelligence scores (both groups scored within the average range).

Youth with short-term mental health problems whose status remained unchanged had a more external locus of control than those whose status improved. Belief in the efficacy of one's own actions was a significant correlate of improvement; reliance on fate, luck, or forces outside one's own control was not.

Discussion

Our findings provide a good example of the wisdom of a recent admonition (Meier 1973) that a comprehensive developmental screening system is useful only if it plugs into practical intervention programs and there is a periodic follow-up to determine the efficacy of treatment.

The Kauai study began before the issue of screening those

under 21 years of age for developmental disabilities became a concern of the federal and many state governments, such as California and Hawaii. Our findings, however, appear to have some relevance to this concern: A cohort of children was periodically screened at birth, in early childhood, and in middle childhood—letters with suggestions for follow-up, where indicated, went to their parents and, with parental consent, diagnostic information was made available to educational, health, and mental health agencies in the community. These agencies were relatively well staffed for the size of the population, were easily accessible, and had a tradition of mutual cooperation.

Yet in what one might call an optimal setting for intervention (if we contrast the small island of Kauai with many big inner cities on the U.S. mainland), only a third of all youth with serious learning or mental health problems in middle childhood received some form of professional help, and less than half of those who did improved between the ages of 10 and 18. This is the aspect of our findings that makes one pause for some serious reflection about the extent and efficacy of intervention in later childhood and adolescence.

Lest we lose our perspective, however, let us remember that the majority of the youth at risk sought and obtained the counsel of their peers, older friends, and parents, and were able to cope quite effectively with temporary crises in childhood and adolescence: Six out of ten among those in need of short-term mental health services (the majority of the childhood behavior problems) reached the threshold of adulthood with increased competence and coping skills.

There is a striking consistency between our findings of a differential improvement rate for different groups of youth at risk (LD, LMH, SMH) in our multiracial sample on Kauai in the 1970s and three major reports in the literature that deal with different historical time spans, different ethnic groups, and different cultures (Levitt 1971; Robins 1966, 1970; Shepherd et al. 1971).

While the impact of treatment during middle childhood and adolescence was relatively slight, parental attitudes had a major impact on improvement among *all* youth with childhood learning and behavior problems, a finding supported by the British survey of childhood mental health (Shepherd et al. 1971) and Masterson's study of adolescents in turmoil (1967).

That not only the mother but also the father plays a predominant role in contributing to the improvement or worsening of his offspring's learning or behavior problems was quite apparent in the responses of the Kauai youth to the 18-year interview. Complementary evidence can be found in an excellent review on the father and the child's mental health by Lynn (1974) and the few studies (Gluck et al. 1964; D'Angelo and Walsh 1967) which have included the father as a focus of treatment.

Of all sources of acknowledged help, peer friends surpassed both parents and professionals in acceptability among the youth on Kauai, most notably to the youth with long-term mental health problems. Offer (1969) noted a similar trend among a group of high school boys representing a "modal" group, ranging between psychopathology and superior adjustment. His boys sought reassurance about themselves among their peers and searched for an interpretation of their behavior. Offer comments that they were good amateur psychologists. The implications for a constructive use of peer counselors in intervention programs for children and youth is clear. Its effectiveness has already been demonstrated in hard-core black poverty areas on the mainland (Roen 1971) and in the use of student companions to children at risk for learning or behavior problems (Cowen 1973).

Differences between improved and unchanged youth at risk appear to be related not only to the presence of parental or peer support but also to communication skills and belief in the efficacy of one's own action, including hard work and persistence. We know from other studies (Coleman 1966; Lefcourt, 1966) that this belief is related to class and caste status.

Socioeconomic status did not affect the *improvement* rate of those with learning disabilities and serious mental health problems who had been exposed to both biological and early environmental stress (though it did affect the *prevalence* rate). However, there was a tendency for more middle-class than lower-class children with short-term mental health problems to improve spontaneously without professional intervention, a trend also found in the British survey of childhood mental health (Shepherd et al. 1971).

The overwhelming majority of the youth with serious learning and behavior problems on Kauai (four out of five) came from cultural backgrounds different from the professionals in the community agencies, who were predominantly Japanese or Caucasian. We can only wonder about possible discrepancies in professional practice and the expectations of the youthful clients and their parents. Levitt (1971) has hypothesized that such disharmony may well contribute to the poor treatment outcomes reported for acting-out and delinquent children.

The concluding remarks from a recent review of the effectiveness of early childhood intervention programs appear also valid in the discussion of intervention in behalf of older children and youth: "A fuller appreciation of the 'cultural differences' as opposed to the 'deficit' model might greatly increase the success of intervention programs with respect to both achievement gains and the maintenance of a positive cultural identity. . . . Whether the results are judged a success or failure may depend on how problems of subcultural patterns of behavior are considered and included in the design and application of intervention programs" (Horowitz and Paden 1973:393).

We turn in the next chapter to a discussion of subcultural differences in achievement orientation and socialization among the different ethnic communities on Kauai.

CHAPTER 11
Subcultural Differences

And if there are not many such scales of value in the world, there are at least several, one for evaluating events near at hand, another for events far away; aging societies possess one, young societies another, unsuccessful people another. The divergent scales of values scream in discordance and daze us, and so that it might not be painful we steer clear of all other values, as though from insanity, as though from illusion, and we confidently judge the whole world according to our own home values.

Alexander Solzhenitsyn
from his acceptance speech for
the Nobel Prize in Literature, 1970

In our previous book, *The Children of Kauai* (1971), the chapter on ethnic differences was but one of a dozen, yet it attracted a great deal of attention. In it we reported differences in infant mortality rates, rates of infant development, school achievement, and patterns of cognitive skills among the five ethnic groups on the island. We also related our findings among the children at ages 2 and 10 to the educational stimulation and the language styles transmitted by their families.

Those interested in differences focused on the lower mean scores found among some of the subcultures on Kauai on developmental tests in infancy and on the different patterns of mental abilities displayed in middle childhood. Because we reported these *differences* (as well as the similarities among the different ethnic groups), some assumed that we subscribed to a deficit model of cognitive and language development. Few noted our strong plea at the end of chap. 10 that it was time to expand our interdisciplinary efforts to learn more about the cognitive and affective development of children from cultures other than our own, since the world these children will inherit is overwhelmingly nonwhite and has a non-Western cultural heritage (Werner et al. 1971:123).

The plea of the present chapter may perhaps go again unheeded, but we would like to state it this time at the beginning: We subscribe to a *difference*, not a deficit, model of human development; we recognize the need for a delicate balance between personal and cultural identity in a pluralistic society such as the United States, but we also see the need for the acquisition of certain patterns of behavior (among them the skills of reading, writing, and speaking Standard English) to survive in a technological society that changes at ever-increasing rates of speed.

Two recent reviews, one on social class and child development by Deutsch (1973) and the other on the effectiveness of environmental intervention programs by Horowitz and Paden (1973), come to similar conclusions about the importance of a balance between the acquisition of cognitive skills needed and valued by the larger culture and the maintenance of affective values which preserve a positive cultural or personal identity.

Since a number of social class and ethnic differences to be reported in this chapter deal with communication skills—and we have already seen in Chapter 10 the importance of these skills in contributing to mental health in adolescence—we offer here a passage from Deutsch that aptly summarizes our view on subcultural language differences:

> Whether the ghetto residents indigenously speak separate dialects or not, it seems that economic advancement—even survival—in a technological society demands that they acquire the prevalent dialect used in the daily life of the culture. It is one thing to classify languages of tribes living encapsulated existences within their own economies and to maintain a scrupulous impartiality on a value scale with respect to drawing comparisons between such groups on the basis of their language.
>
> It is quite another matter to attempt to maintain the same attitude with respect to subgroups which are . . . interdependently entwined economically with the larger culture which surrounds them. In the latter case the tools of *any* trade that the subgroup members will elect will include understanding of and use of the dominant language system. (Deutsch 1973:271-272)

This chapter focuses first on subcultural differences in verbal communication skills as measured by the SCAT and STEP, group tests of scholastic aptitude and achievement routinely used in Hawaii's high schools during the time of our follow-up in adolescence. We then present interpersonal variables that appear related to differences in achievement orientation and socialization among the different ethnic communities on the island. We close this chapter with a look at both similarities and differences among adolescents from different ethnic groups and different social classes who have successfully combined high scholastic achievement with a positive identification with their own subcultures.

Differences on the SCAT and STEP

In Tables 35 and 36 we present the mean scores and standard deviations on the SCAT, grades 8 to 10 and 12, for youth from five ethnic groups on Kauai. They are the Japanese, ethnic mixtures of predominantly Japanese-Filipino parentage (offspring of older Filipino fathers and younger Japanese mothers), the Filipinos, the Hawaiians and part-Hawaiians, and the Portuguese, whose ancestors came originally from the Azores to work on Kauai's sugar plantations (see Chapter 2).

Although there were a few (3 percent) Anglo-Caucasians among the cohort of 1955 births, all from middle-class or upper-middle-class families, only two Haole males (both scoring at or above the national norm) were attending Kauai's public high schools; the remainder were in private schools on other islands.

Within each ethnic group, we show a breakdown of means and standard deviations on the verbal, quantitative, and total scales of the SCAT, at each grade level, by social class. The SES rating combines information on the father's occupation, income level, steadiness of employment, and condition of housing (see Chapter 3). It is based primarily on the father's occupation: Professionals, proprietors, and managers make up the "upper" class; skilled, trade, and technical workers the "middle" class; and semiskilled and day laborers the "lower" class.

We used two-way analyses of variance to compare the main effects of social class (upper and middle vs. lower) and ethnicity and possible interaction effects for all SCAT scales in grades 8 to 10 and 12. The results show a striking resemblance to our earlier findings on the Primary Mental Abilities Test (PMA) during our 10-year follow-up (Werner, Simonian, and Smith 1968).

There were significant *social class* differences, favoring

middle- and upper-class children, on all three SCAT scales, both at the beginning and end of high school, in each of the five ethnic groups. Social class differences *increased* from grade 8 to grade 12 (with the exception of the verbal scale on the SCAT).

There were also significant *ethnic group* differences on all subtests of the SCAT, both in grades 8 to 10 and grade 12. Ethnic group differences operated independently from social class (interaction effects were not significant for any subtest at any grade), as they had previously on the PMA (Werner et al. 1971). Ethnic group differences, though significant, were not as pronounced as social class differences.

Among the five ethnic groups, the Japanese continued to

Table 35 Mean Percentile Scores and Standard Deviations of Five Ethnic Groups by SES on the SCAT (Grades 8 to 10), 1955 Cohort

Ethnic Group	SES	SCAT Verbal		SCAT Quantitative		SCAT Total	
		$\overline{X}$	SD	$\overline{X}$	SD	$\overline{X}$	SD
Japanese	U	49.0	25.6	71.3	25.9	60.3	26.2
(N=179)	M	53.9	25.1	60.3	27.4	57.1	26.0
	L	42.5	23.8	47.5	30.2	42.9	26.2
Filipino	U	28.5	.7	49.5	46.0	37.5	23.3
(N=91)	M	44.1	22.2	34.4	24.9	38.1	24.8
	L	30.1	20.3	35.8	24.3	30.5	21.6
Hawaiian and part-							
Hawaiian	U	84.0	—	81.5	9.2	64.5	5.0
(N=96)	M	36.6	24.1	39.8	27.6	36.5	26.0
	L	28.7	19.9	26.8	21.2	25.1	19.2
Ethnic mixture	U	64.3	31.4	72.3	39.5	68.8	37.9
(N=72)	M	36.8	25.6	36.6	28.3	35.1	27.1
	L	31.6	24.2	29.2	22.0	29.0	24.8
Portuguese	U	39.3	35.0	47.3	31.5	43.3	35.2
(N=38)	M	42.6	23.9	39.8	30.0	38.9	26.5
	L	25.5	26.1	23.1	20.6	22.5	24.3
Results of Two-Way ANOVA	F	df	p	F	df	p	F	df	p
Ethnicity	3.64	4	<.01	7.06	4	<.01	5.78	4	<.01
SES	19.25	1	<.01	18.84	1	<.01	22.68	1	<.01
Interaction	.18	4	NS	1.20	4	NS	.36	4	NS

rank consistently above the other ethnic groups (as they had at age 10). Their mean scores were at the national average of 50 on the verbal scale and above the national norm on the quantitative scale. Mean scores of the other ethnic groups tended to be about one standard deviation below the mean of the Japanese and *decreased* from beginning to end of high school on the verbal scale. The rank order of the ethnic groups in this cohort remained constant across time (from grades 4 to 8–10 to 12), tests (from PMA to SCAT), and socioeconomic levels.

The distribution of the means should not obscure the overlap in scores that exist among youth from different subcultures. For any two ethnic groups, there were students in one who scored

Table 36 Mean Percentile Scores and Standard Deviations of Five Ethnic Groups by SES on the SCAT (Grade 12), 1955 Cohort

Ethnic Group	SES	SCAT Verbal		SCAT Quantitative		SCAT Total	
		$\overline{X}$	SD	$\overline{X}$	SD	$\overline{X}$	SD
Japanese	U	55.2	28.2	67.6	31.5	62.1	30.5
(N=156)	M	52.3	27.1	66.1	28.0	59.7	27.4
	L	36.2	21.7	49.6	29.5	42.2	24.4
Filipino	U	33.0	—	80.0	—	54.0	—
(N=79)	M	33.8	25.3	34.0	27.8	32.5	27.9
	L	29.1	23.3	35.6	25.8	30.8	24.9
Hawaiian and part-Hawaiian	U	66.0	—	79.5	19.1	76.0	8.5
(N=73)	M	38.6	25.7	43.8	28.7	43.3	28.1
	L	20.6	18.5	23.2	22.2	18.7	18.5
Ethnic mixture	U	55.3	40.1	72.3	34.0	63.7	43.1
(N=55)	M	40.3	25.3	38.7	30.0	38.1	29.1
	L	27.5	22.9	26.8	28.0	25.8	25.3
Portuguese	U	42.0	36.3	51.7	41.3	47.3	39.6
(N=33)	M	30.1	16.8	43.5	29.4	37.5	23.5
	L	23.7	24.5	22.0	21.0	22.1	22.0

Results of Two-Way ANOVA	F	df	p	F	df	p	F	df	p
Ethnicity	2.82	4	<.05	5.04	4	<.01	3.92	4	<.01
SES	15.86	1	<.01	23.23	1	<.001	24.20	1	<.001
Interaction	.84	4	NS	1.75	4	NS	1.34	4	NS

higher than some students in the other. Among youth in the lower-SES class, there were some who scored higher than other youth in the upper- and middle-SES levels.

It is interesting to note that the variance in the test scores was greater among the middle and upper middle class than among the poor in *all* ethnic groups on the island, a finding similar to that reported by Scarr-Salapatek (1971) from a study of black and white twins in Philadelphia. She argues from her findings that biological differences in ability may manifest themselves conspicuously in people (of all races and cultures) who develop in favorable and stimulating environments and remain undisclosed in adverse and suppressive environments.

In Tables 37 and 38 we present the means and standard deviations for the same five ethnic groups on the STEP, both for grades 8 to 10 and grade 12. Again, there were significant *social class* differences in all ethnic groups on all tests (reading, mathematics, and writing), and the social class differences *increased* from the beginning to the end of high school.

There were also significant *ethnic group* differences on the STEP operating independently from social class, but they were not as pronounced. The rank order of the ethnic groups was nearly the same on the achievement test as on the scholastic aptitude test. The Japanese consistently had mean scores at the national average (reading) or slightly above (mathematics and writing); mean scores of the other ethnic groups tended to be lower and *decreased* on the writing and reading scales of the STEP from the beginning to the end of the high school period.

In sum: Deficits in verbal skills, i.e., in understanding, reading, and writing Standard English, already noted (at age 10) were *cumulative* and increased for most lower-class youth during their high school years on Kauai, with the exception of the Japanese. The implications for more limited educational and vocational choices for these youth in a complex technological society are clear, no matter how strong and positive their cultural identity may be.

Our findings on Kauai agree with reports from another neighbor island, Hawaii (Dixon et al. 1968), and from the analysis of a 20 percent random sample of all students attending public high schools in the state of Hawaii who were tested in grade 10 and retested in grade 12 (Stewart et al. 1967). Both studies found consistent and highly significant ethnic variations on the SCAT (verbal and quantitative scales) and various achievement tests, favoring the Japanese (and in the case of the statewide sample the Chinese as well). The only other large-scale study of ability and achievement on the U.S. mainland that included Oriental-Americans (Coleman 1966) found that they scored at or above the Caucasian mean on achievement test scores throughout grade school and high school and surpassed them in mathematics achievement, a trend reflected in the higher mean scores on the SCAT quantitative and STEP mathematics scales among the Japanese youth on Kauai.

In previous publications (Werner, Simonian, and Smith 1967, 1968; Werner et al. 1971) we discussed some of the differences in language style and the quality of educational stimula-

Table 37   Mean Percentile Scores and Standard Deviations of Five Ethnic Groups by SES on the STEP (Grades 8 to 10), 1955 Cohort

Ethnic Group	SES	STEP Reading		STEP Mathematics		STEP Writing	
		$\overline{X}$	SD	$\overline{X}$	SD	$\overline{X}$	SD
Japanese	U	55.2	31.4	61.2	27.9	65.8	26.4
(N=179)	M	57.5	24.7	56.7	26.1	65.2	25.6
	L	49.5	25.7	47.5	23.6	57.7	27.5
Filipino	U	15.0	7.1	47.0	46.7	31.0	38.2
(N=91)	M	31.1	26.7	35.1	28.2	48.6	30.7
	L	35.6	22.2	33.9	18.9	44.3	28.4
Hawaiian and part-							
Hawaiian	U	55.0	32.5	67.5	17.7	61.0	12.7
(N=98)	M	39.4	24.8	42.7	26.5	38.1	29.0
	L	27.0	19.8	30.2	18.2	34.1	23.7
Ethnic mixture	U	69.5	37.2	73.0	36.3	78.0	32.2
(N=72)	M	32.1	29.6	34.2	23.3	44.4	30.2
	L	32.3	25.6	34.4	23.9	37.3	26.4
Portuguese	U	50.0	36.5	46.7	34.8	53.7	43.5
(N=39)	M	41.7	23.8	38.0	22.2	50.5	25.9
	L	25.3	26.0	32.2	15.2	27.5	24.8
Results of Two-Way ANOVA	F	df	p	F	df	p	F	df	p
Ethnicity	6.71	4	<.01	5.69	4	<.01	7.31	4	<.01
SES	9.84	1	<.01	9.65	1	<.01	11.92	1	<.01
Interaction	1.23	4	NS	.43	1	NS	1.39	4	NS

tion transmitted by the families that might account for the persistent subcultural differences on scholastic aptitude and achievement tests. Later on in this chapter we take a look at differences in cultural expectations, parental socializing styles, and the relative strength of affiliative vs. achievement motivation among the different ethnic communities on the island.

An appropriate link between the cognitive and affective domain is an intrapersonal variable that is strongly related to achievement: the locus of control dimension. It measures the degree to which a person believes that a behavioral event is contingent upon his or her own actions. Those who believe that events

Table 38   Mean Percentile Scores and Standard Deviations of Five Ethnic Groups by SES on the STEP (Grade 12), 1955 Cohort

Ethnic Group	SES	STEP Reading		STEP Mathematics		STEP Writing	
		$\overline{X}$	SD	$\overline{X}$	SD	$\overline{X}$	SD
Japanese	U	54.1	29.7	64.0	27.2	59.1	28.4
(N=164)	M	51.5	26.3	63.1	26.3	57.1	26.2
	L	41.6	25.7	43.1	23.3	42.7	27.3
Filipino	U	40.5	—	84.0	—	42.0	—
(N=81)	M	30.9	33.2	45.2	24.7	41.9	25.7
	L	30.0	23.7	35.5	24.1	34.8	26.2
Hawaiian and part-Hawaiian	U	45.5	35.5	79.0	14.1	45.5	17.7
(N=76)	M	38.1	27.1	41.0	23.9	36.3	24.7
	L	28.0	22.1	27.5	21.3	27.8	22.6
Ethnic mixture	U	78.0	26.9	73.0	31.2	65.3	51.5
(N=59)	M	36.5	26.5	43.0	22.5	43.3	28.4
	L	31.8	27.7	32.7	24.7	30.4	25.3
Portuguese	U	43.7	36.1	44.5	3.5	42.3	38.6
(N=33)	M	34.7	19.8	38.1	23.6	42.6	35.7
	L	19.8	25.5	28.7	16.2	21.9	18.9
Results of Two-Way ANOVA	F	df	p	F	df	p	F	df	p
Ethnicity	2.48	4	<.05	3.85	4	<.01	3.32	4	<.05
SES	12.04	1	<.01	19.71	1	<.01	18.22	1	<.01
Interaction	.15	4	NS	.71	4	NS	.71	4	NS

happen to them as a result of fate, luck, or other factors beyond their control are called "externals"; "internals" are characterized by the belief that their own actions determine the positive or negative reinforcement they receive. In most of the reported cross-cultural studies, groups whose social position is one of minimal power, either by class or race, tend to score higher in the external control direction (Lefcourt 1966). What differences, if any, do we find among Kauai's youth?

Differences on the Locus of Control Scale

In Table 39 we present the mean scores and standard deviations of youth from the same five ethnic groups (Japanese, Filipino, Hawaiian and part-Hawaiian, Portuguese, and other ethnic mixtures), by sex and social class, on the Novicki Locus of Control Scale (Novicki and Duke 1972).

The rank order of the five ethnic groups on Kauai on the Locus of Control Scale corresponds closely to their rank order on tests of scholastic aptitude and achievement. While none of the ethnic groups on the island appeared quite as internally motivated as the Anglo-Caucasians, the Japanese were the least external, especially the females, and the Portuguese were the most external, especially the males.

Upper-middle-class members of ethnic groups that rank generally low on the socioeconomic ladder of the island (Portuguese, Hawaiians, and other ethnic mixtures) were the least external, followed by the middle-class Japanese. Upwardly mobile Filipinos were the most external. Both ethnic and social class differences, however, were only suggestive: A two-way analysis of variance failed to show significant main or interaction effects for these two variables.

Our results, though only suggestive, support the findings of Coleman (1966) that both Caucasian and Oriental-American high school students on the mainland appeared to have greater faith in their own control of the environment than blacks, Native Americans, Mexican-Americans, and Puerto Ricans. Achievement or lack of achievement appeared closely related to what the youth believed about their environment—whether they believed the environment would respond to reasonable efforts or whether they believed it was merely random and immovable. We have seen the same self-fulfilling prophecy at work among the pregnant teen-

Table 39 Mean Scores and Standard Deviations of Five Ethnic Groups by Sex and SES on Novicki Locus of Control Scale (Grades 11 and 12), 1955 Cohort

	Total (N=361)		Japanese (N=137)		Filipino (N=75)		Hawaiian and part-Hawaiian (N=67)		Other Mixtures (N=52)		Portugese (N=29)	
	$\overline{X}$	SD	$\overline{X}$	SD	$\overline{X}$	SD	$\overline{X}$	SD	$\overline{X}$	SD	$\overline{X}$	SD
Total	13.49	4.67	12.75	4.54	13.87	5.08	13.96	4.45	13.87	4.42	14.38	4.92
Sex												
Male	13.83	4.78	12.87	5.10	14.61	4.91	14.12	3.84	13.70	4.24	17.50	4.84
Female	13.13	4.52	12.58	3.72	13.18	5.21	13.79	5.02	14.16	4.81	12.74	4.21
SES												
Upper			43.65	3.66	15.00	—	12.00	2.83	6.00	1.00	10.50	3.54
Middle			12.18	4.32	14.31	5.82	13.26	4.37	5.57	4.01	14.55	3.17
Lower			13.30	5.10	13.75	5.00	14.43	4.55	13.86	4.05	14.75	5.96

agers and youth with short-term mental health problems who improved (or failed to improve)—on their own—during adolescence
(see Chapters 8 and 10). Though the concept of locus of control
may not be a unitary phenomenon, scores on the Novicki scale appear to have a strong relationship to school achievement and improvement in status for problem youth in adolescence.

Differences on the CPI

Tables 40 and 41 show the means and standard deviations of
males and females from the three largest ethnic communities on
Kauai (Japanese, Filipinos, and Hawaiians) on the 18 subscales of
the California Psychological Inventory. Brislin et al. (1973:237) in
their recent handbook of cross-cultural research methods state:
"By any reasonable cross-cultural criteria the CPI ranks as the
most well-known and prolifically used objective personality test."
It has been used in a series of cross-cultural studies in Africa,
Asia, Europe, and Latin America (Brislin et al. 1973), most
recently in studies of socialization and delinquency among
Japanese students (Gough et al. 1968) and studies of achievement
orientation among black, Native American, and Mexican-
American high school students in the United States (Benjamin
1969; Mason 1967).

The 18 CPI subscales cluster in four classes: (1) measures of
poise, ascendency, self-assurance, and interpersonal adequacy; (2)
measures of socialization, maturity, responsibility, and intrapersonal structuring of values; (3) measures of achievement potential
and intellectual efficiency; and (4) measures of intellectual and interest modes. Since the CPI subscales are intercorrelated, a discriminant function analysis was used to examine differences in the
responses of the three ethnic groups, by sex, to the inventory.

Two discriminant functions accounted for the variability
among the females of Japanese, Filipino, and Hawaiian descent at
the $p < .0001$ and $p < .03$ level of significance respectively. The
two discriminant functions that emerged from the comparison of
the CPI responses of the males did not differentiate the three
ethnic groups at a statistically significant level (p values were
$< .24$ and $< .28$ respectively), but there were similarities in trends
between the responses of the men and the women from the
different descent groups.

Among the women in the three major ethnic groups, discriminant function 1 accounted for 68 percent of the variance. The CPI scales with the highest loadings on this function were:

1. Responsibility (+.51): identifies persons of conscientious, responsible, and dependable disposition and temperament (high score)
2. Communality (+.49): indicates the degree to which a person's response corresponds to the modal (common) pattern established for the inventory (high score)
3. Well-being (+.45): identifies persons who minimize their worries and complaints and who are relatively free from self-doubt and disillusionment (high score)
4. Flexibility (+.44): indicates the degree of flexibility and adaptability of a person's thinking and social behavior (high score)
5. Socialization (+.42): indicates the degree of social maturity the person has attained (high score)

Table 40   Means and Standard Deviations of Japanese, Filipino, and Hawaiian Females at Age 18 of the CPI

Subscale	Japanese (N=59)		Filipino (N=43)		Hawaiian and part-Hawaiian (N=38)	
	$\overline{X}$	SD	$\overline{X}$	SD	$\overline{X}$	SD
Do	20.7	5.5	23.2	5.8	21.8	5.8
Cs	13.6	3.4	13.6	4.1	13.2	3.8
Sy	19.1	5.1	21.0	4.4	20.3	4.8
Sp	28.9	4.9	31.1	4.8	31.3	4.6
Sa	18.8	4.1	19.5	3.4	19.1	4.3
Wb	28.4	6.6	24.6	6.8	25.0	6.8
Re	26.1	4.9	24.4	5.5	20.8	5.7
So	35.6	6.4	32.4	6.6	32.0	7.0
Se	22.1	7.5	20.7	6.9	20.7	6.7
To	14.5	4.9	12.1	5.4	12.1	4.6
Gi	12.1	4.7	12.4	5.0	13.3	5.5
Co	25.2	2.3	23.5	3.5	22.4	5.4
Ac	20.0	5.0	21.0	6.2	18.7	4.7
Ai	14.7	3.7	13.1	4.1	13.1	5.0
Ic	28.9	5.1	27.3	6.7	25.6	7.7
Psych	7.3	2.6	7.4	2.5	7.9	2.3
Fx	8.8	3.5	6.7	3.1	6.9	4.5
Fe	25.0	3.3	26.4	13.4	22.2	4.2

Table 41   Means and Standard Deviations of Japanese, Filipino, and Hawaiian Males at Age 18 on the CPI

Subscale	Japanese (N=76)		Filipino (N=34)		Hawaiian and part-Hawaiian (N=35)	
	$\overline{X}$	SD	$\overline{X}$	SD	$\overline{X}$	SD
Do	21.3	5.4	21.3	3.0	20.1	3.8
CS	13.6	3.4	14.3	3.7	13.4	3.5
Sy	19.4	4.8	20.7	4.8	19.6	3.4
Sp	30.9	5.3	31.1	5.2	29.8	4.9
Sa	18.4	3.5	18.4	3.2	17.6	4.0
Wb	26.1	6.7	24.5	6.6	24.3	6.3
Re	24.0	4.6	21.3	3.9	19.8	4.3
So	32.2	6.0	31.2	6.3	28.7	6.1
Se	21.6	6.2	20.6	5.6	20.7	5.0
To	13.8	4.3	12.3	4.8	13.0	3.3
Gi	12.8	4.8	13.8	4.9	13.3	4.8
Co	21.8	4.9	19.9	4.9	19.6	5.7
Ac	19.3	4.8	19.3	4.3	18.3	3.8
Ai	14.1	4.3	12.9	3.8	12.5	2.9
Ic	28.1	5.9	26.3	6.2	26.7	4.8
Psych	8.8	2.6	8.6	2.5	8.3	1.7
Fx	8.9	3.6	9.3	3.6	8.0	2.6
Fe	18.6	11.2	17.0	3.6	15.8	3.2

6. Tolerance (+.40): identifies persons with permissive, accepting, and nonjudgmental social beliefs and attitudes (high score)

7. Social presence (−.40): assesses factors such as poise, spontaneity, and self-confidence in personal and social interaction (low score)

8. Intellectual efficiency (+.32): indicates the degree of personal and intellectual efficiency the person has attained (high score)

As a group, Japanese adolescent women on Kauai scored higher on this discriminant function than either Filipino or Hawaiian adolescent women. Adjectives characteristic of high scorers are:

Is responsible, serious about duties and obligations; dependable, conscientious

Is predictable; stands at the midpoint on most topics and issues

Has a good fund of energy; not a worrier or complainer; optimistic

Is adaptable and flexible

Is able to accept rules and authority; has good judgment; is socially mature

Accepts others and their beliefs; is open-minded; values tolerance

Is resourceful; efficient; gets things done; *but* lacks somewhat in self-confidence and spontaneity

Discriminant function 2 accounted for 32 percent of variance among the adolescent women in the three major ethnic groups. The CPI scales with the highest loadings on this function were:

1. Responsibility (+.47): identifies persons of conscientious, responsible, and dependable disposition and temperament (high score)
2. Femininity (+.43): assesses femininity of interests (high score)
3. Achievement via conformance (+.35): identifies those factors of interest and motivation which facilitate achievement in any setting where conformance is a positive behavior (high score)
4. Dominance (+.22): assesses factors of leadership ability, dominance, persistence, and social initiative (high score)

As a group, Filipino adolescent women on Kauai scored higher on this discriminant function than Japanese adolescent women, who in turn scored higher than Hawaiian adolescent women. Adjectives characteristic of high scorers are:

Is responsible; serious about duties and obligations; dependable, conscientious

Works well in situations having clear-cut rules and regulations with strong need for achievement; finds it easy to do well under supervision

Is gentle in manner, nurturant; *but* also strong, resolute, dominant, persistent

Differences among the males of the three major ethnic groups on the CPI were not as pronounced as among the females. Discriminant function 1 accounted for 54 percent of the variance among the adolescent males in three the major ethnic groups. The CPI scales with the highest loadings on this function were:

1. Socialization (+.55): indicates the degree of social maturity the person has attained (high score)
2. Communality (+.50): indicates the degree to which a person's responses correspond to the modal (common) pattern established for the inventory (high score)
3. Responsibility (+.49): identifies persons of conscientious, responsible, and dependable disposition and temperament (high score)
4. Achievement via independence (+.47): identifies those factors of interest and motivation which facilitate achievement in any setting where autonomy and independence are positive behaviors (high score)

As a group, Japanese adolescent males tended to score somewhat higher on this discriminant function than Filipino adolescent males, who in turn scored somewhat higher than Hawaiian adolescent males. Adjectives characteristic of high scorers are:

Is able to accept rules and authority; has good judgment; does not behave in a rash or thoughtless manner; socially mature
Is predictable; moderate on most topics and issues
Is responsible; serious about duties and obligations; dependable and conscientious
Has strong need for achievement and works well in situations stressing independence and initiative; does not need direction or guidance

Discriminant function 2 accounted for 46 percent of the variance among the adolescent males from the major ethnic groups on Kauai. The CPI scales with the highest loadings on this function were:

1. Flexibility (+.32): indicates the degree of flexibility and adaptability of a person's thinking and social behavior (high score)
2. Sociability (+.29): identifies persons of outgoing, sociable, participative temperament (high score)
3. Tolerance (−.28): identifies persons with permissive, accepting, and nonjudgmental beliefs and attitudes (low score)

4. Capacity for status (+.24): measures the personal qualities and attributes which underlie and lead to status (high score)

As a group, Filipino adolescent males tended to score somewhat higher on this function than either Japanese adolescent males or Hawaiian adolescent males. Adjectives characteristic of high scorers are:

Likes change and variety; seeks new experiences and adventures; is adaptable and flexible

Is sociable, outgoing; likes social activity

Is ambitious, tends to get ahead; gives the impression of being successful

Is also somewhat aloof, wary, and judgmental in attitudes

The result of our discriminant function analyses of the CPI appear to reflect differences in the social position and social mobility among the youth from the three major ethnic communities on Kauai and the degree to which each of the three subcultures, especially the females, identify with the dominant American society.

Though the CPI is based on folk concepts that are said to be "aspects and attributes of interpersonal behavior found in all cultures and societies" (Gough 1969:57), there appear to be differences among the youth of the three subcultures in the degree to which their responses correspond to the common or modal pattern established for the inventory (originally standardized on Caucasian mainland samples).

When we look at the communality scale, we see that Japanese-American youth, as a group, score higher on this dimension than Filipino-Americans, who in turn score higher than the Hawaiian and part-Hawaiian youth. In each ethnic group, females tend to score higher than males.

Of the three subcultures, the Japanese-American youth, coming from predominantly middle-class homes, appear to value those personality characteristics that maintain their status in an achievement and efficiency-oriented society, but without losing their respect for rules and authority and their sense of obligation to others significant in their lives. This seems to be especially true for the Japanese-American females. Their highest scores, as a group, are on measures of socialization and responsibility and measures of achievement potential and intellectual efficiency (at some cost in spontaneity). They seem secure enough to afford a moderate point of view on most issues and to be tolerant of differing beliefs and opinions.

The Filipino-American youth of Kauai, coming from predominantly lower-middle and lower-class homes, respond, as a group, like an upwardly mobile subculture. They have identified enough with the predominant culture to strive for status in that society, but the emphasis for the Filipino-American adolescents tends to be on the *social* aspects of "getting ahead," which is particularly striking among the females. In comparison with the Japanese and the Hawaiian-American youth, Filipino-American adolescents tend to score higher on measures of self-assurance and interpersonal adequacy, especially the women. Filipino-American females score high on traditional concepts of femininity, but also high on dominance.

As a group, the Hawaiian and part-Hawaiian adolescents, coming from the bottom of the socioeconomic ladder, display a somewhat different response pattern on the CPI than most youth from the other two subcultures. Their responses tend to be least like the common or modal pattern, defined by the middle-class Caucasian standardization group, on which the CPI norms are based. They are more in tune with a concept of personality that values spontaneity and self-confidence in personal and social interaction for women (Hawaiian adolescent girls, as a group, score higher on social presence than women from the other two subcultures) and traditional masculine interests and pursuits for the men (Hawaiian adolescent men, as a group, score higher on this dimension than males from the other two subcultures).

The differences in response to the CPI, however, appear not to be unique for the three ethnic communities on Kauai but can be found among other subcultures on the mainland which differ in social status and social mobility.

There is an interesting similarity between the pattern of responses of the Japanese-American youth on Kauai and the CPI scores of academically successful black high school students living in a midwestern ghetto community. Benjamin (1969) found that academically successful black females had significantly higher mean scores than unsuccessful black females on the following CPI subscales: responsibility, socialization, communality, and achievement via conformance. Successful black males had, in addition, higher mean scores than unsuccessful black males on intellectual efficiency and a sense of well-being.

Among culturally disadvantaged junior high school students on the U.S. West Coast, Mexican-American males whose families counted for economic support on the success of their sons scored high on the responsibility, tolerance, and intellectual efficiency scales of the CPI, as did the Japanese-American high school seniors on Kauai (Mason 1967).

In contrast, the responses of the Native American students were very similar to those of the Hawaiian youth on Kauai. Most of the Native American youth had been exposed to the debilitating effects of family disorganization, to the weakening of tribal organizations, and to strong local prejudice. They were, like the Hawaiians, "strangers in their own land" (McNassor and Hongo 1972).

Other investigators (Dixon et al. 1970; Fenz and Arkoff 1962; Meredith and Meredith 1966), using different personality inventories with high school and college students in urban settings of Hawaii such as Honolulu and Hilo, have reported that in all ethnic subgroups the women were more homogeneous in their responses and appeared more assimilated. We found this same trend in rural Kauai and thought it appropriate to close this chapter with a look at the antecedents of achievement orientation among Hawaiian, Japanese, and Filipino women in our cohort who combined scholastic success with a strong identification with their own family and subculture.

Differences in Achievement Orientation

The antecedents of achievement-oriented behavior have recently become the focus of extensive cross-cultural research (LeVine 1970). Most studies of achievement motivation have concentrated on Western youth (in the United States, Latin America, and Europe), and almost all have dealt with boys. The majority have focused on McClelland's one-drive achievement model (N Ach); N Ach has been defined as an intrinsic drive for excellence and success, with little concern for the approval of others, acquired through independence and early mastery training by a supportive caretaker, usually the mother (McClelland 1961).

McClelland's achievement model well suits the mainstream of American culture. However, achievement motivation may not be found in the same social and psychological context in every culture. According to DeVos (1968, 1973), achievement orientation can have two role components, *instrumental* and *expressive*.

Instrumental role behavior is performed as a means to an end rather than for the immediate satisfaction inherent in the act itself. Expressive role behavior gains satisfaction in the act itself or in the relationship in which the behavior is expressed.

While McClelland's theory, based on Western samples, stresses the instrumental aspects of achievement orientation, there is need for additional research with non-Western samples to explore the role of *expressive* factors in achievement. Most of the research done so far with Oriental or Polynesian boys tends to favor the expressive factors in achievement (Caudill and DeVos 1961; Kubany et al. 1970; Slogett et al. 1970).

By far the largest amount of research has been done on the achievement orientation of Japanese-Americans (Arkoff and Leton 1966; Berrien et al. 1967; Horinouchi 1967; Kitano 1961, 1969; Meredith 1965; Meredith and Meredith 1966). They have been educationally and vocationally more successful than many other ethnic groups that have come to the United States from Asia. Their success appears to be due to the fact that the Japanese immigrants had values that coincided with the majority Western culture, although they were motivated by expressive rather than instrumental role behavior (Caudill and DeVos 1961). Japanese immigrant mothers socialized their nisei children toward high need affiliation (N Aff) and a concern with the opinion of others and cooperation which conflicts with the Western notion of individualistic N Ach. However, the instrumental component may come to play a more important part among the more acculturated sansei (third-generation Japanese-Americans). In a recent study, Slogett et al. (1970) found that sansei adolescent men exhibited significantly more instrumental than expressive themes in their response to the Thematic Apperception Test than Filipino and Hawaiian youth.

In the traditional Hawaiian home, the complex family system and tight peer relationships tend to foster the child's dependency on the group (Boggs 1968; Gallimore 1969; Gallimore et al. 1974; Gallimore and Howard 1968). The group, in turn, emphasizes harmony and cooperation, which tends to conflict with competition and achievement in a Western-oriented school system. Traditional patterns of childrearing in the Philippines seem very similar to Hawaiian values and attitudes toward raising children (Guthrie and Jacobs 1966; Nydegger and Nydegger 1966). Filipino parents also stress the need to contribute to the family and they value peer acceptance. Two recent studies that have focused on the achievement-oriented behavior of Hawaiian and Filipino-American adolescent men have found expressive themes as their prime motive for achievement (Kubany et al. 1970; Slogett et al. 1970).

Although women among Hawaii's major ethnic groups appear more acculturated and achievement-oriented than men (Meredith and Meredith 1966; McNassor and Hongo 1972), little is known about the antecedents of their achievement orientation. We therefore decided to take a look at the aspiration levels and antecedents of achievement orientation among the Japanese-American, Hawaiian-American and Filipino-American women in the 1955 cohort who ranked among the top ten in their respective ethnic groups on measures of scholastic aptitude and academic achievement (Fricker and Werner 1976).

All the women had grades reflecting above average achievement in college preparatory classes (B+ or better) and scores in the top quartile of the SCAT and STEP in grades 10 and 12. The 10 Japanese-American women came from middle-class homes with smaller families (average number of siblings, three) and better-educated parents (mean years of schooling for father, 12; for mother, 13.5). The 10 Hawaiian and 11 Filipino women came from homes with low incomes, large families (mean number of siblings for Hawaiians, 6.0; for Filipinos, 5.0), and parents who, as a rule, had not graduated from high school (mean years of schooling for Hawaiian fathers, 9.0; for Filipino fathers, 7.9; mean years of schooling for Hawaiian and Filipino mothers, 9.7).

Specific questions were selected out of the 18-year interview (see Appendix 4) to ascertain the level of educational and vocational aspirations of the young women, the antecedents of their achievement orientation, and the strength of expressive and instrumental components in their achievement orientation. In addition, a comparison was made of the responses of their mothers on the family interview conducted during the follow-up at age 10. The interview included information on the interests and activities in the home, the values placed by the family on education, the work habits emphasized in the home, and opportunities provided to explore the larger community. Though all the women from each ethnic group were highly intelligent and had achieved high standards of scholastic success in a competitive Western school system, their future educational and vocational aspirations were different. Most of the Japanese and Filipino women aspired to a bachelor's degree or more, while most of the Hawaiian women were content with high school graduation or some additional training at the local community college (chi square=10.62; df=2; $p < .005$).

More high-achieving women of Japanese and Filipino descent had definite plans for a college education and a career, while the Hawaiian women were split between marriage and the pursuit of additional education or work (chi square=4.70; df=2; $p < .10$). Significantly more high-achieving women of Japanese and Filipino descent aspired toward professional careers such as engineering, journalism, law, management, medicine, politics, and research; more high-achieving women of Hawaiian descent were content with traditional female occupations such as clerk, nurse, secretary, or tourist entertainer (chi square=7.80; df=2; $p < .025$).

The Filipino women had the highest levels of educational and vocational aspirations among the three groups. Although they came as a rule from very poor homes with large families and had parents who had not graduated from high school, 8 out of 10 planned to do graduate work, enter a professional career, and combine a career with having a family.

All high-achieving women viewed their father as easy to talk to and felt he had a moderate to strong influence on them. The fathers had stressed academic goals and wanted their daughters to extend their education beyond high school. However, some significant differences between the ethnic groups appeared in the daughters' perception of their mothers. All daughters of Hawaiian and Japanese descent described their mothers positively, compared with only half the Filipino women (chi square=10.84; df=2; $p < .01$). Daughters from Hawaiian and Japanese homes found it easier to talk to their mothers than daughters from Filipino homes (chi square=6.24; df=2; $p < .05$). Most mothers from Japanese homes, but even more from Filipino homes, expected their daughters to receive a college degree, whereas most Hawaiian mothers only expected some training past high school (chi square=8.20; df=2; $p < .025$).

The three groups differed significantly (chi square=9.69; df=2; $p < .025$) as to which parent they chose as main model for themselves. The Hawaiians were equally divided between their mothers and their fathers. The Japanese women modeled after their mothers or both parents. Filipino women modeled after their mothers exclusively.

Early responsibility training is considered an important antecedent of achievement motivation (McClelland 1961). From the mothers' interviews it was possible to see how much and what type of responsibility had been placed on their daughters at the age when achievement orientation tends to crystallize. All girls had been delegated chores around the house by the time they were 10 years old. There was a tendency for mothers and daughters in Hawaiian and Filipino families to share more home-based activities, such as baking, cooking, sewing, and cleaning house; more Japanese mothers and daughters shared recreational activities outside the home, including shopping trips and visits to the library (chi square=5.21; df=2; $p < .10$).

More Hawaiian and Filipino mothers were pleased with and stressed expressive personality traits in their daughters, such as eagerness, helpfulness, being good-natured, obedient, popular, being a good listener. A higher proportion of the Japanese-American mothers were pleased with and stressed their daughters' school achievement (chi square=4.84; df=2; $p < .10$). Instrumental characteristics mentioned by the daughters as their strong points were aggressiveness, hard work, persistence, and intellectual interests. Expressive traits valued were being good-natured, understanding, friendly, honest, patient, generous, and empathetic. There were no significant differences among the three groups in the frequency with which instrumental or expressive traits were mentioned as assets or as goals for self-improvement. The students' descriptions of worries were also divided between instrumental concerns, such as grades, school achievement, and success in a career, vs. expressive concerns, such as the needs of family and friends or the opinion of others. There were no significant differences among the three groups in the frequency of these concerns. All three groups of high-achieving women scored in the internal direction on the Locus of Control Scale, manifesting a strong belief in the control of their fate.

Our results indicate that the mothers were the most influential role models for their high-achieving daughters. In each of the three ethnic groups the mothers of the high-achieving women had, as a rule, more education than the fathers—a trend also noted by McNassor and Hongo (1972) among high-achieving Hawaiian adolescent men. The Hawaiian and Japanese daughters appeared to have a close, positive relationship with their mothers, whereas the Filipino daughters had a more ambivalent relationship.

The Hawaiian mothers' and daughters' commitment to traditional sex roles and success in homemaking and childrearing seemed to provide a consistent framework for close identification. Both the Japanese mothers and their daughters valued high educational and occupational achievement; their commitment to the same goal lends itself to a congruent relationship.

The dynamics of the Filipino mother-daughter relationship appears to be more ambiguous. The ambivalence may be due to an incipient conflict between sex role ideologies of mothers and daughters and the coexistence of high dominance and femininity in both (see CPI results). A study conducted on the mainland with Caucasian samples found that mothers with traditional sex role ideologies had ambivalent relationships with their career-minded daughters who had more contemporary sex role ideologies (Lipman-Blumen 1972). Even though it is desired by her mother, the Filipino-American daughter's pursuit of a professional career may cause deterioration or tension in the traditional, closely knit family system. The potential for conflict for these young women and their parents is mitigated, however, by a balance between their commitment to educational and vocational achievement and their desire to please their family and kin who value education.

The positive message these young women leave for other youth on the island and for minority youth on the mainland is that one can acquire the cognitive skills needed and valued by the larger American society without sacrificing affective ties with family and ethnic identity.

The importance of these affective ties needs to be recognized in any community intervention program designed to assist youth from different subcultures who were not as fortunate as these young women in solving the developmental problems of childhood and adolescence. Other writers (Gallimore and Howard 1968; McNassor and Hongo 1972) have commented on the Hawaiian preference for personal as opposed to impersonal relationships, for cooperation rather than competition. Operating in the context of personal relationships is both familiar and comfortable for many of the youth and families of Oriental and Polynesian descent. Hence professional and agency personnel who try to deliver services on a personal and supportive basis will likely be the most successful.

Lest we be tempted to call many of these youth and their families "deprived," we need to be reminded that deprivation is a relative concept. What industrialized man gains in an increased ability to abstract, to categorize, and to control, he may well lose in decreased spontaneity and sensitivity to the uniqueness of people and events.

In the Hawaiian spirit of *kokua* ("cooperation") professionals, parents, and youth might learn from each other by reasoning together and being sensitive to each other's feelings and needs. For, as Thomas Griffith (1974) wrote in a *Time* essay:

> The stubborn American belief in equality does not depend on a false claim of similarity among men when their differences are real. Instead, it argues for a broader test in judging each person's qualities. By deploying his own range of qualities as best he can, each man frames his own dignity and asserts his right to look any other man squarely in the face.

CHAPTER 12
On the Threshold of Adulthood

So far, our discussion has focused primarily on youth who have been subjected to biological and/or environmental stress and who subsequently developed serious learning and behavior problems in childhood and adolescence.

We would be remiss, however, if we did not also share with our readers some of the biographical data we were able to obtain on the present status and future plans of nearly 90 percent of the cohort of 18-year-olds on Kauai (*N*=560).

Much of the literature on adolescence and young adulthood has had a crisis orientation: The data on which it is based have been drawn primarily from youth in conflict with themselves or with society at large (King 1972). Lest we lose our perspective, however, it is important also to take a look at groups of normal adolescents, representing the whole range between psychopathology and superior adjustment, as was done on the mainland by Offer (1969).

It has been customary, lately, to speak and write about the "gap between the generations," about the failure of the American public school system, about the tendency of youth to turn away from cherished parental values and abandon the pursuit of education and occupational success in favor of a search for fulfillment through drug use and sexual freedom, in short, to drop out of the system.

Many of these impressions have been gleaned from a look at small, economically and educationally privileged groups of Caucasian youth or from studies of hard-core poor, both black and white, in the inner cities of the mainland. We found few of these symptoms among the youth of Kauai.

Our population consisted of the children and grandchildren of immigrants who left the poverty of their Asian homelands to find a better future in the cane fields of Hawaii. For most, this meant a semiskilled or unskilled job on the plantations. Many intermarried with the local Hawaiians who, under the impact of successive waves of newcomers, lost many lives, much land, and many remnants of their own culture.

While their children came of age, statehood came to Hawaii; and tourists and the impact of the space age reached even this seemingly remote island. Throughout all these changes, most parents, though poor by material standards, kept their dream of the "good life," the hope for a better education and a better job for their children. Was this dream in vain? We do not think so, but readers must judge for themselves.

Educational Status and Plans

Ninety-seven percent of the cohort of 18-year-olds had graduated from high school; only 3 percent dropped out without receiving a graduation certificate. This is a remarkably low rate of educational waste and a tribute to the efforts of the public school system to reach potential dropouts through work motivation classes, special classes for pregnant teenagers, off-campus classrooms, and Outreach counselors. It is also a tribute to the steadfast belief of parents and youth in the value of education. Few of the immigrant parents, with the exception of the Japanese, had themselves been high school graduates. In 1950, the median years of schooling for the mothers' generation of Kauai women 25 years or older was eight grades; median years of schooling for the fathers' generation of Kauai men 25 years or older was only six grades, reflecting the presence of the older immigrant sector of the population, especially the Filipinos.

Academic success had been mentioned by the youth in the interviews at age 18 as the foremost goal of *both* their fathers and their mothers (36 percent of the fathers gave it top priority, as did 37 percent of the mothers). About a third (33 percent) of the fathers and the mothers (29 percent) looked forward to some training beyond high school for their sons and daughters; a fourth hoped that their offspring would graduate from college (26 percent of the fathers, 25 percent of the mothers). They were not disappointed by their children.

About one-fifth (19 percent) of the 18-year-olds planned to pursue some technical, vocational, or business training beyond high school. Another fifth (21 percent) were about to enroll in the local community college, a branch of the University of Hawaii that had grown from 250 to 1,000 students in the eight years between our 10-year and 18-year follow-up. Nearly a third (29 percent) of the high school graduates in this cohort planned to attend a four-year college, either the Univerity of Hawaii in Honolulu or university campuses on the mainland, mostly on the West Coast (California, Washington). Thirteen percent hoped to attend graduate school. Many had worked during the summers to save money for college; some had taken on loans to free their parents from a considerable expenditure that might involve not only tuition but travel to and room and board on the mainland. Those heading for college, if they came from poor homes, considered a step-by-step approach: the first two years at the Kauai Community College, the next two years at the University of Hawaii, and then graduate school in Honolulu or on the mainland.

Thus the local community college was perceived as an important gateway to higher education and occupational advancement for many youth from poor homes who would be the first college-educated generation in their family. It is worth noting here that Hawaii is the only state in the union without autonomous local school districts. Money raised through income and excise taxes is portioned out equally to every student, whatever community college or public school she or he may attend.

Vocational Status and Plans

About one-half of the 1955 cohort had had some work experience during high school or were working by the time they had reached age 18, either in the sugar plantations, in the tourist industry, or in small businesses. Many of the girls had paid babysitting jobs. There were some interesting differences between the occupational levels of their parents and the vocational aspirations of Kauai's youth at age 18, some 80 percent of whom had definite occupational plans or at least some fairly specific criteria for the choice of an occupation.

Only 2 percent of the parents' generation held professional jobs. In contrast, 7 percent of their offspring planned to go into professions (law, dentistry, medicine) and another 5 percent into teaching.

Only 7 percent of the parents were engaged in semiprofessional, proprietory, or managerial jobs. In contrast, 38 percent of the youth planned to go into business, the most popular vocational choice among the cohort. An additional 4 percent aimed for managerial jobs in wholesale or retail business.

Thirty-five percent of the fathers were employed in skilled trade or technical jobs. In contrast, only 5 percent of their offspring planned to go into skilled trades (carpenter, mechanic, plumber). Ten percent of the youth, mostly girls, aimed for clerical and secretarial jobs; 15 percent of the boys hoped to join the police or the military service.

Forty-two percent of the fathers worked in semiskilled jobs and 14 percent in unskilled and day labor jobs in the plantations and, lately, the tourist industry. In contrast, only 3 percent of their offspring wanted to go into the tourist industry, but 14 percent chose plantation work. Only a small minority (6 percent) were undecided or chose deliberately to drop out (8 percent).

The vocational aspirations of the youth seem to reflect a desire for upward mobility—from the lower and lower middle class to the middle class and from the middle class to the upper middle and upper class. There appears to be one exception: The proportion choosing to work in the sugar plantations was approximately the same for both the fathers' and the sons' generations.

There is certainly no indication that these youth have rejected parental beliefs in occupational advancement and the advantages of middle-class life. There is also no indication that most of the youth, given a choice, would like to opt out of the system. If anything, their desire for upward mobility may be somewhat unrealistic given the options open for them on the island and the changes that have taken place in the last decade (see Chapter 2) and are foreseeable in their adult future. For instance, it is highly unlikely that there will be much room for an expansion of owner-operated small businesses on Kauai or, for that matter, elsewhere on Hawaii or the mainland. On the other hand, there is an increasing need for people to work in the growing tourist industry (apparently not particularly favored by the youth), in federal and state government, and in skilled trades. Thus there may be a need for some redirection of vocational objectives that could be achieved by counseling in the senior year in high school or freshman year in community college or university or by extending vocational guidance services by other community agencies.

Views on Marriage, Children, and Work

At the time of the 18-year follow-up, 6 percent of the 1955 cohort were married; an additional 3 percent were engaged and planned to be married shortly. Eight percent of the adolescent women had given birth to one or more babies or were pregnant. Another third had a very steady, exclusive arrangement with one partner. The remainder expressed an interest in heterosexual activities and participated in parties and group activities, but a sizable number, after having had a steady boyfriend or girlfriend during the early years of adolescence, felt now that it was too early for them "to get tied down," that they needed to find themselves first. This was especially true for those planning to go to college or get some additional vocational training, and it applied to the young women in this sample as well as the men. Typical were remarks like this one from a male: "We were going steady for a while, but I didn't want to be tied down. We're just friends. I just want to enjoy being by myself, see if I can handle it." Or this from a female: "I have a boyfriend, he is older than I. We've been going together for about two years. ["Do you have serious plans with him?"] Yes, but not until I am older. He knows that I have to continue [business] school and wait a while and pay my loan off. I don't want to get married until I am a little older and more mature."

About two-thirds of the young women interviewed planned to work first and marry later; about one-third wanted to marry first. Only one-fourth were interested only in marriage and not in outside work. The overwhelming majority of the young women (three out of four) planned to combine work and marriage, possibly a reflection of the spirit of women's liberation but also a necessity on an island where the cost of living is high (rates of married women working are higher in Hawaii than on the mainland). Eighty percent of this group planned to combine work, marriage, and motherhood. The group was about equally divided between those who planned to work regardless of the age of their children, those who planned to work when their children entered school, and those who wanted to work when their children left home.

Clearly there is a need for some counseling of these young women and their partners, including the teenage mothers (see Chapter 8) to help them fulfill their multiple roles in the most satisfying way for themselves and their families.

Parental Influence

Contrary to the popular myth of the generation gap, the interview responses of Kauai's youth showed a great deal of parental influence on their offspring, not only in matters of education and vocation but also in matters of morality and personal goals for their future. Two out of three youth interviewed identified strongly with their father and three out of four with their mother.

Two-thirds felt that their father had exerted a moderate to strong degree of influence on them, as had their mother. Most chose their mother as the person most likely to discuss problems with at home, and the majority felt that she listened and tried to understand them as a separate individual worthy of respect. A slightly lower proportion, still the majority, felt the same way about their father's understanding. Two-thirds found their father supportive of most things they wanted, as they did their mother. Most felt that they had been taught morality by parental example and their parents' teaching. Relationships with siblings were reported to be smooth for the majority of the 18-year-old youth, though some reported spats in their early teens. Most had found a strong feeling of security in their family. A happy, successful marriage had priority among their future goals and achievements (ahead of success in a career or job), surely a compliment to their own parents and family.

Coping with Problems

The majority of the youth in the 1955 cohort were able to cope effectively with their problems with the help of parents, peers, and older friends. Only one out of five of all youth in the cohort had some contact with the police during their adolescence, and less than one out of ten with other social agencies in the community. Multiple agency contacts were heavily concentrated on the relatively small number of youth who had serious learning disabilities and mental health problems in childhood (see Chapters 5 to 8).

Most common in the cohort were minor health problems (20 percent) such as allergies, respiratory problems, and, for the boys, minor injuries in sports. Only 4 percent reported having major physical problems during this period.

About 60 percent of the 18-year-olds interviewed saw the need for improvement in themselves. The smallest proportion were concerned with physical attributes (4 percent), some (7 percent) wanted to improve their school performance, and nearly half (45 percent) saw some need for improvement in personality traits.

Peer friends were by far the most popular source of help in coping with their personal problems (35 percent), followed by older friends (including siblings, relatives, boyfriend's or girlfriend's parents [20 percent]) and their own parents (12 percent). Two-thirds of the youth interviewed sought help from these three sources of support; only a third turned to professionals, such as counselors (11 percent), teachers (7 percent), psychiatrists, psychologists, social workers (7 percent), or ministers (2 percent). Nearly three out of four youth interviewed (73 percent) had never thought of any need for psychotherapy; 15 percent considered it, but did not go; 12 percent went occasionally or regularly. The majority (some 80 percent) felt that the support and counsel they received from friends and parents helped a lot. They were able to cope by dealing directly with their problems and sharing their feelings with others.

Views on Social Issues

The late sixties and early seventies saw the advent of the Haole hippies on Kauai. Their search for serenity and inner awareness by the use of drugs and their rejection of established values brought social changes and conflicts which were completely outside the experience of the island youth. The harassment of one group by the other and the use of drugs became a not uncommon experience. Drugs are now easily available and there is a great deal of freedom on the youngsters' part in making their choice about their use (see Chapter 2). We were therefore interested to get the views of the 18-year-olds who had lived through these social changes in their teens on three issues of major concern to them and the community: drug use, premarital sex, and race relations.

Nearly two-thirds of the youth interviewed (64 percent) favored some restriction of drugs by *society at large*; one-fourth (24 percent) in this group believed they should be outlawed altogether. The remainder were split between those who had no opinion on society's control of drugs (20 percent) and those who thought the use of drugs was each person's individual choice (14 percent). There were some differences between problem and control youth on this issue: More of the problem youth had no opinion on the matter; more of the control youth favored restriction and outlawing of drugs.

When asked about their *personal* position on the use of drugs, 56 percent stated that they did not and would not use any drug whatsoever; 21 percent indicated that they use or might use marijuana, but nothing else; only 3 percent stated that they used or might use other drugs, including hard drugs (that latter response came only from the new problem cases in adolescence). The others were uncertain or had no position on the personal use of drugs. The proportion among the 18-year-olds on Kauai who responded in the affirmative regarding the use of marijuana is nearly identical to that found (24 percent) in a survey of adolescent drug use among high school students on the West Coast (Johnson et al. 1971).

Typical of the comments received were these:

> It was really bad for the kids. I heard that even in elementary school, they're starting to do it now. Parents think there's no hope already as the kids are getting too rough and out of hand. [*Question*] Talk to them about it to make them stop before they get into it—make the laws more strict. [*Question*] I used to use drugs. [*Question*] Grass, pills—now I don't, I don't think I would again. Kids get into it for kicks and to ease the pain in their minds.

> I'm actually afraid of them—when you see your friends and read about people. I'm really afraid I might be somehow addicted to it. . . . I really think whatever the legislature or government does won't do as much help as what a person himself decides.

> It doesn't bother me—some drugs I can see why they don't make it legal and some I cannot. [*Question*] I can't see anything wrong with marijuana. [*Question*] I use it, once in awhile. [*Question*] Drinking is OK too—just that you have to have the money.

> Guess I feel society should control it more, but I can't say how. One way though I feel is if a person wants to use it, let him use it, it's his life.

The youths' attitudes toward premarital sex were certainly more liberal, but not more promiscuous, than their parents' generation. Fifty-six percent condoned premarital sex relations: Of these, 42 percent thought it was all right when the partners were close and 14 percent thought it was necessary and natural when you loved each other. The remainder were clearly against premarital sex (18 percent), were uncertain (13 percent), or did not want to discuss the issue (13 percent). The wide range of attitudes can be seen in the following comments:

> Well, it's up to the boy and the girl what they think about it—if they feel right about it, up to them if they want to do it or not.

> It depends on how *you* feel about it. I don't think anything's wrong with it. The way I felt was I told myself I was going to stay clean till I met somebody I really really loved.

> OK as long as they do it in a respectful way—not just something to use and pull aside and talk about. [*Question*] I think I've said enough.

> I don't know—lots of people say it's OK and up to them and all that stuff. [*Question*] I don't know.

> I haven't really thought about it—it doesn't throw me anyplace.

Among the youth interviewed, opinions about race relations varied from those indicating no prejudice existed to those viewing it as a serious problem. Approximately one out of four felt there were no problems; one out of five thought there was some prejudice; and one out of three viewed the problem as moderate to severe. There were no apparent differences between youth with or without serious learning and behavior problems in the range of opinions expressed. Only about 60 percent of the youth interviewed could verbalize the direction the prejudice took. Over half of these stated that prejudice existed against Haoles—particularly the mainland Haole newcomer. This opinion resembled that expressed in the McNassor and Hongo study (1972), where the greatest resentment was toward the hippies "who stole our waves." Resentment against new immigrants from the Philippines and local Japanese was about even (in 20 percent of those noting direction of prejudice), while blacks bore the brunt of 6 percent of the directed opinions. Many noted that there was a tendency for youth to band together by race or neighborhood but this did not constitute a problem. Examples of the range of statements follow:

> There's none on Kauai—didn't feel it in high school—I went to the states and in the service noticed people were prejudiced.

Not in school here—but I myself am prejudiced against blacks, the way they act—the attitude—they act too good or whatnot—I guess if I had a close friend who was black, I'd understand them.

First of all I was prejudiced. [*Question*] Against Japanese and Haoles, the kind that came from the mainland. The reason was I felt they were acting like the know-it-alls, like they were in a different class than us. I can get along with them—anyone that played sports with me.

There's some, but not too much. I'm not bothered by it. It's a hassle about mainland Haoles. I was born here. I'm against mainland ones too—they're just invading. They destroyed the mainland and are trying to destroy us. [*Question*] The hotels, surfing, and all, but there is not much we can do about it.

I really think there was more prejudice in school between the Japanese and Haoles and our group—Filipinos, Hawaiians, and Portuguese. More of the Japanese were in Phase IV [grouping by ability and achievement level] and thought they were on a high level and couldn't come down to our level and have some fun. The parents tell their kids not to play with the Filipinos and Hawaiians as they'll teach you to steal—you'll get hurt.

Here I see it [prejudice] plainly. Mostly if you're Japanese, you're always with Japanese friends; if Haole, always with Haoles. There's a few exceptions. [*Question*] The group I'm with has mixed Hawaiian friendships. But if you go into the library, you see a big gang of Japanese talking, and the Haoles and Filipinos segregated. But not to a bad extent, there's not really fighting except at the beaches. [*Question*] Usually the Hawaiians there. I know I'm prejudiced—at least I go along with it, don't buck it, fight the Haole! [*Question*] From surfing. Starts with stealing the waves. . . . The wise guys grab your board. . . . The prejudice is more against newcomers. [*Question*] More based on actions—it all gets back to the "dirty Haole." Mostly the ones born here are OK. It's widespread from school to school. In Honolulu it's not only the Haoles that are hated, but the Japanese too. There's not so much prejudice against the Japanese here as in Honolulu.

Not really much prejudice. As they say, "Kauai is beautiful."

Discussion

Our survey of the 18-year-olds on Kauai agrees with the findings of other recent studies on coping and growth in adolescence (King 1972; Masterson 1967; Offer 1969):

1. Turmoil and conflict appear limited to a relatively small number of youth, most of whom had already shown signs of disturbance in early and middle childhood. The overwhelming majority in our cohort were competent in coping, began to develop a sense of identity, and showed a strong continuity with past experiences.

2. There was little evidence for a generation gap: Fathers and mothers were generally viewed as supportive and understanding by most of the youth. The overwhelming majority of the 18-year-olds chose one or both parents as models and showed a strong sense of continuity with their families in values attached to education, occupational preference, and social expectations.

3. Most adolescents had good relationships with their siblings and turned to them for counsel and emotional support.

4. Although many of the youth saw a need for self-improvement, most had found ways of coping successfully with problems by sharing them with friends and parents and by preparing themselves realistically for the adult future.

Our data on the vocational aspirations of the mostly upwardly mobile youth and their views on social issues of importance to them and their community (drug use, premarital sex, race relations) suggest, however, that there is some need for counseling the "normal" youth—to help them with a realistic choice of vocation in a changing technological world, to inform them about the long-term consequences of using seemingly harmless drugs, to discuss openly the responsibilities involved in sexual freedom, and to find together a way to live peaceably in a multiracial society in which we are all our brother's keeper.

CHAPTER 13
Early Predictors of Problems

This chapter addresses itself to the predictive validity of diagnostic signs from birth records, psychological and pediatric screening examinations, and family interviews at 2 and 10 years. It is intended as a bridge between the concerns of the clinician who is interested in the fate of the relatively small group of children identified as having serious learning or behavior problems by middle childhood and the concerns of the professional whose major interest is in the mass screening of large populations of children for the early identification and prevention of behavior and learning disorders.

How well did each set of variables in this study, the sociological, the biological, and the psychological data, singly or in combination, identify groups of potential problem children? How early was it possible to make significant predictions? Did the predictive validity of our tools vary with outcome, with the sex of the child, with socioeconomic background? These are the questions we attempt to answer in this chapter.

We first present a series of tables that summarize correlations, across time, between predictors at birth, year 1, year 2, and year 10 and problems at ages 2, 10, and 18. We discuss the significance of these findings, with special reference to sex differences, and the likelihood of improved prediction for children from lower-SES homes.

We next present a set of multiple correlations that show the best combinations of predictors which identified children who had low scores on developmental and pediatric examinations at age 2 and children who were diagnosed as mentally retarded or needing placement in learning disability classes or mental health services at age 10.

We then look at predictions across the whole time span of this longitudinal study, from birth, infancy, and middle childhood to age 18, to see how well we were able to predict the likelihood of the occurrence of mental health problems and delinquency in late adolescence.

Finally we isolate a set of variables, some sociological, some biological, some psychological, that appeared to be the most effective in "red flagging" youngsters with potential problems in childhood and adolescence and could be obtained economically from records at birth and in school, from developmental screening in infancy, and from group tests in the early elementary grades.

Predictions of Two-Year Outcomes

Table 42 summarizes the correlations between selected variables from records at birth, as well as maternal ratings of infant behavior at year 1 and the results of the two-year psychological and pediatric screening examinations.* Ninety-six percent of the cohort of 1955 births were given these examinations during our two-year follow up; thus the attrition rate between the beginning of the study and the first follow-up was very low. Of the 320 boys in the 1955 cohort, 23 (7 percent) received Cattell IQs below 80 on the developmental screening examination and 38 (13 percent) were considered to be below normal (slow or defective) in physical development in an independent pediatric examination which consisted of a systematic appraisal of all organ systems (see *The Children of Kauai* chap. 3). Of the 312 girls, 13 (4 percent) scored below 80 on the Cattell Infant Intelligence Scale and 42 (15 percent) were considered to be below normal in physical development

---

*The median age at the time of the pediatric examination was 19½ months; at the time of the psychological examination it was 20 months, with 95 percent of the children examined by age 2. For convenience they are referred to here as the two-year examinations.

by the pediatricians. Thus, while the proportion of boys and girls considered below normal in physical development was comparable, nearly twice as many boys as girls scored low on the developmental examination.

As can be seen in Table 42, predictions from data obtained around birth and maternal infant behavior ratings at year 1 were generally higher for children with Cattell IQ scores below 80 at two years than for those the pediatricians considered below normal in physical development. This was true for both boys and girls. Correlations between data obtained at birth or year 1 and two-year Cattell IQ scores ran generally a little higher for the girls. Correlations between the same set of data and the pediatrician's assessment of physical status at age 2 ran generally a little higher for the boys.

PREDICTORS OF CATTELL IQ BELOW 80

The best single predictor of a low Cattell score at age 2 was the presence of congenital defects at birth. This variable correlated .43 with Cattell IQ below 80 for the boys and .45 for the girls. Predictions from this variable were slightly higher for both boys and girls from homes whose standard of living had been considered low at birth ($r=.49$ for both sexes).

When we combined all information available at birth and infant behavior ratings at year 1, we obtained a multiple R of .59 for the girls and a multiple R of .55 for the boys. Predictions were slightly higher for boys and girls from poor homes (multiple R of .61 for both sexes). A combination of congenital defects, moderate to severe perinatal stress, chronic conditions judged by physicians to be leading to minimal brain dysfunction, and a low standard of living and maternal education (eight grades or less) were the most powerful predictors for the girls ($R=.58$). A combination of congenital defects, chronic conditions leading to minimal brain dysfunction, a low standard of living at birth, and low ratings of infant activity level and social responsiveness by the mother at year 1 were the most powerful predictors for the boys ($R=.53$).

PREDICTORS OF PHYSICAL STATUS BELOW NORMAL

The best single predictors of below normal physical status at age 2 were the presence of congenital defects at birth for the boys

Table 42 Predictions of Two-Year Outcomes from Data Available at Birth and Year 1

Predictor	Cattell IQ Below 80		Physical Status Below Normal	
	Males (N=23) r	Females (N=13) r	Males (N=38) r	Females (N=42) r
Mother's education	.14	.25	.20	.15
Standard of living at birth	.18	.21	.12	.17
Psychological trauma during pregnancy	.002	.06	.10	.02
Perinatal stress	.08	.28	.19	.21
Chronic conditions leading to MBD	.12	.10	.09	.16
Congenital defects	.43	.45	.26	.06
Birthweight	.04	.06	.20	.18
Difficulty of labor	.08	.07	.05	.05
Twin designation	.06	.00	.12	.19
Baby not affectionate	.16	.09	.09	.10
Baby's activity level	.23	.04	.20	.01
Distressing habits of baby	.04	.07	.07	.02

($r=.26$) and the presence of moderate to severe perinatal stress for the girls ($r=.21$). Predictions from these variables were slightly higher for children from poor homes, yielding $r=.29$ for the girls and $r=.27$ for the boys. When we combined all information available at birth and the infant behavior ratings at year 1, we obtained a multiple R of .47 for the boys and a multiple R of .37 for the girls. Multiple correlations were higher for children from poor homes ($R=.56$ for the boys, $R=.43$ for the girls).

A combination of congenital defects, moderate to severe perinatal stress, birthweight below 2,500 grams, low activity level of the baby at year 1, and little education of the mother were the most powerful predictors for the boys ($R=.46$). A combination of moderate to severe perinatal stress, chronic conditions leading to minimal brain dysfunction, birthweight below 2,500 grams, twin birth, and low standards of living and maternal education were the most powerful predictors for the girls ($R=.36$).

IN SUM: Biological insult at or around birth, especially to the central nervous system, coupled with a poor standard of living at birth, was predictive of poor developmental outcomes in early childhood. Maternal behavior ratings of low activity level and low social responsiveness (baby not cuddly or affectionate) added to the predictive power for the boy infants; a low level of maternal education added to the predictive power for the girl infants.

Predictions of 10-Year Outcomes

In *The Children of Kauai* (chap. 9) we addressed ourselves to the predictive value of the two-year pediatric and psychological screening examinations in forecasting the likelihood of significant physical handicaps, low school achievement, and low intelligence test scores at age 10. We reported then that the earlier diagnoses for children with significant physical handicaps were largely confirmed at age 10. The Cattell IQ at age 2 proved to be the best predictor of IQ and achievement at age 10 (with $r=.40$ for PMA IQ and $r=.44$ for achievement level).

We found a high positive correlation ($R=.80$) with IQ at age 10 for children with Cattell IQs below 80 when we combined their developmental score on the psychological examinations with the pediatrician's rating of developmental status arrived at independently. A combination of low socioeconomic status and retarded development noted by the pediatricians or psychologists for children at age 2 more accurately predicted later serious school achievement problems than did either examinations or environmental ratings alone.

In this section we extend some of the findings reported then by examining the early factors predictive of mental retardation, learning disabilities, and the need for mental health services at age 10. It should be noted that attrition rates for the 1955 cohort during the 10-year follow-up were still relatively low: We were able to obtain 10-year data on 90 percent of the original cohort. Of the 320 boys in the cohort, 15 were diagnosed as mentally retarded, 14 needed placement in a learning disability class, 14 needed long-term mental health services, and 30 needed short-term mental health services. Among the 312 girls, 10 were diagnosed as mentally retarded, 8 needed placement in a learning disability class, 11 needed long-term mental health services, and 30 needed short-term mental health services.

In every category of "poor" outcomes at age 10, with the exception of children needing only short-term mental health services, there were proportionately more boys than girls.

PREDICTORS OF MENTAL RETARDATION

As can be seen from Table 43, predictions from data obtained in infancy were generally higher for the diagnostic category "mental retardation" than for the other criteria at age 10 and ran higher for the girls than for the boys. The best single predictor of mental retardation at age 10, for both sexes, was a Cattell IQ score below 80 at age 2. It correlated .46 with a diagnosis of mental retardation for the boys and .52 for the girls. When we combined all variables available from our data at birth, year 1 and year 2, we obtained a multiple R of .66 for the girls and a multiple R of .57 for the boys. (Predictions for low-SES children improved only for the boys with a multiple R of .62.)

A combination of low Cattell IQ score, low Vineland SQ score, low rating of psychological status at age 2, presence of congenital defects, and a mother with little education were the most powerful predictors for the girls (R=.65). A combination of low Cattell IQ and low rating of psychological status, with little family stability at age 2 and a mother with little education who had experienced psychological trauma during pregnancy (a variable assessed during the first phase of the study) were the most powerful predictors for the boys (R=.54).

Table 43 Predictions of 10-Year Outcomes from Data Available at Birth and Infancy: Mental Retardation and Learning Disabilities

Predictor	Mental Retardation		Learning Disability	
	Males (N=15) r	Females (N=10) r	Males (N=14) r	Females (N=8) r
Mother's education	.21	.27	.06	.06
Standard of living at birth	.22	.22	.09	.25
SES at 2	.19	.12	.07	.17
Family stability at 2	.19	.12	.09	.14
Psychological trauma during pregnancy	.17	.05	.05	.05
Perinatal stress	.02	.18	.08	.07
Chronic conditions leading to MBD	.13	.08	.07	.06
Congenital defects	.19	.17	.02	.03
Birthweight	.05	.01	.02	.08
Difficulty of labor	.03	.003	.09	.09
Twin designation	.04	.30	.04	.01
Baby not affectionate	.09	.09	.10	.004
Baby's activity level	.19	.09	.15	.05
Distressing habits of baby	.01	.001	.05	.08
Cattell IQ	.46	.52	.12	.35
Vineland SQ	.33	.33	.12	.06
Psychologist's assessment of intellectual development	.36	.31	.14	.31
Psychologist's assessment of psychological status	.18	.13	.04	.12
Pediatrician's assessment of physical development	.37	.26	.06	.23

IN SUM: A Cattell IQ score below 80 at age 2 appeared to be predictive of a diagnosis of mental retardation at age 10. The predictive power of the results of the infant test increased with the addition of information on biological factors (presence of congenital defects) in the girls and with the addition of data reflecting early emotional instability in the home (low family stability, psychological trauma during pregnancy) for the boys.

PREDICTORS OF LEARNING DISABILITY

As in the case of mental retardation, predictions from data obtained in infancy were higher for girls considered in need of placement in a learning disability class at age 10 than for the boys in the same diagnostic category.

For the girls, the best single predictor of learning disability at age 10 was again a Cattell IQ score below 80 at age 2 ($r=.35$). For the boys, the best single predictor was the mother's rating of the baby's high activity level at year 1 ($r=.15$). A combination of all data available at birth and in infancy yielded a multiple R of .49 for the girls and a more modest multiple R of .27 for the boys.

Predictions increased slightly for children from poor homes (multiple R of .53 for the girls, multiple R of .32 for the boys). A combination of Cattell IQ below 80, presence of congenital defects and chronic conditions judged by physicians to lead to minimal brain dysfunction, difficult labor, birthweight below 2,500 grams, and a low standard of living and maternal education were the most powerful predictors for the girls in this group ($R=.46$). A combination of moderate to severe perinatal stress, ratings of high activity level and social responsiveness at year 1, and a home rated low in family stability at age 2 were the most effective predictors for the boys ($R=.24$).

IN SUM: Predictive in both sexes were a combination of biological insult to the central nervous system around birth and an early home environment low in stability. Infant temperamental traits nonrewarding for the mother appeared more frequently in boys who were later diagnosed as learning disabled than in girls.

PREDICTORS OF MENTAL HEALTH NEEDS

In general, correlations between our data in infancy and outcomes at age 10 were higher for boys and girls in need of long- term mental health (LMH) services than for children considered in need of short-term mental health (SMH) services only. However, by comparison with previous sets of predictions they were more moderate than the correlations reported between birth data and developmental problems at year 2 (low Cattell IQ, below normal physical development) and between infancy data and diagnoses of significant physical handicaps, mental retardation, or serious learning problems at age 10.

LMH Children. The multiple R between a combination of infancy data and the diagnosis of need for long-term mental health services at age 10 was $R=.37$ for the girls and $R=.36$ for the boys. Multiple correlations increased slightly for children of the poor, to $R=.40$ for the girls and $R=.38$ for boys.

As can be seen from Table 44, the best single predictor for the girls was a low standard of living at birth ($r=.18$) and for the boys it was a low SES rating of the home at age 2 ($r=.18$).

A combination of low standard of living, maternal education, and family stability, birthweight below 2,500 grams, moderate to severe perinatal stress, distressing habits of baby and high activity level noted by the mother at year 1, and a low rating of the infant's intellectual and psychological status at age 2 were the most effective predictors for the girls ($R=.36$). A combination of low socioeconomic status, low birthweight, moderate to high perinatal stress, presence of congenital defects and chronic conditions judged by physicians to lead to minimal brain dysfunction, and a maternal rating of low social responsiveness at year 1 and low social maturity at age 2 were the best predictors for the boys ($R=.35$).

IN SUM: In both sexes an interaction between biological impairment around birth, a low standard of living and distressing or non-rewarding temperamental traits in infancy appeared to be moderately predictive of long-term mental health problems in middle childhood.

SMH Children. Our lowest correlations between infancy data and outcomes at age 10 were for the largest group of problem children, those considered in need of short-term mental health services at age 10. This was true for both boys and girls, though our predictions improved somewhat for the children of the poor. We know from our follow-up in adolescence that the overwhelming majority of these children reacted to temporary stress in middle childhood and improved spontaneously without intervention by the time they had reached the threshold of adulthood.

As can be seen in Table 44, there were very few statistically

Table 44 Predictions of 10-Year Outcomes from Data Available at Birth and Infancy: Mental Health Needs

Predictor	LMH Children		SMH Children	
	Males (N=14) r	Females (N=11) r	Males (N=30) r	Females (N=30) r
Mother's education	.17	.14	.17	.01
Standard of living at birth	.17	.18	.09	.01
SES at 2	.18	.12	.05	.09
Family stability at 2	.09	.16	.10	.04
Psychological trauma during pregnancy	.02	.02	.01	.03
Perinatal stress	.04	.10	.04	.01
Chronic conditions leading to MBD	.13	.07	.09	.05
Congenital defects	.07	.08	.01	.04
Birthweight	.15	.06	.05	.05
Difficulty of labor	.03	.02	.05	.08
Twin designation	.04	.01	.06	.02
Baby not affectionate	.14	.02	.17	.01
Baby's activity level	.10	.07	.07	.002
Distressing habits of baby	.01	.14	.05	.03
Cattell IQ	.13	.10	.02	.03
Vineland SQ	.001	.06	.06	.08
Psychologist's assessment of intellectual development	.16	.06	.11	.07
Psychologist's assessment of psychological status	.05	.10	.04	.08
Pediatrician's assessment of physical development	.01	.10	.08	.002

significant correlations between earlier data and 10-year outcomes for these children. The best single predictors for the boys, though barely significant, were a low level of maternal education and a low level of social responsiveness at year 1 (baby rated not affectionate by mother) ($r=.17$). For the girls, none of the earlier variables correlated to a statistically significant degree with 10-year outcome.

A combination of all data available from birth through year 2 yielded a modest multiple correlation for the girls ($R=.23$) and a slightly higher one for the boys ($R=.30$). For both sexes, predictions improved slightly for children from poor homes: The multiple R for girls from low-SES homes rose to .29; for boys it rose to .35.

A combination of a low level of maternal education and family stability in the home at age 2, a high level of activity and nonresponsive behavior in the infant (baby not affectionate), and a Cattell IQ below 80 was most predictive of later short-term mental health problems in boys ($R=.28$). A combination of low social maturity and low rating of psychological status coupled with a low socioeconomic status and low family stability at age 2 was the most effective set of predictors for girls ($R=.20$).

IN SUM: The relatively low correlations between our data at birth, year 1, and year 2 and the presence of short-term mental health problems in middle childhood confirm our impression, gained from our follow-up data in adolescence, of the transient nature of most of these behavior problems, especially among girls (see Chapter 7). The likelihood of the appearance and persistence of these problems was, however, greater for the children of the poor.

Predictions of 18-Year Outcomes

Table 45 summarizes the correlations between selected variables from birth, year 1, year 2, and year 10 and two types of "deviancy" in late adolescence: serious mental health problems and delinquency. Serious mental health problems by age 18 included youth (23 males, 47 females) who had been sent to the Hawaii State Mental Hospital or local hospitals for mental health reasons, youth who had made one or more suicide attempts, youth who were or had been recently under treatment as outpatients of the Kauai Community Mental Health Center, and youth who, on the basis of our 18-year interview data, had been judged to have seri-

Table 45 Predictions of Problems in Adolescence from Data Available at Birth, Year 1, Year 2, and Year 10

Predictor	Delinquency by 18		Serious Mental Health Problems by 18	
	Males (N=77) r	Females (N=26) r	Males (N=23) r	Females (N=47) r
Mother's education	.16	.18	.20	.07
Standard of living at birth	.16	.12	.21	.22
SES at 2	.12	.10	.13	.31
Family stability at 2	.19	.09	.13	.06
SES at 10	.20	.26	.20	.25
Educational stimulation at 10	.23	.19	.27	.25
Emotional support at 10	.16	.23	.29	.20
Congenital defects	.09	.24	.02	.14
Baby's activity level at 1	.03	.02	.16	.03

Cattell IQ at 2	.04	.38	.07	.13
Vineland SQ at 2	.02	.14	.02	.04
Pediatrician's assessment of physical development at 2	.05	.14	.09	.06
PMA IQ at 10	.24	.26	.24	.29
PMA verbal score at 10	.24	.20	.22	.27
PMA reasoning score at 10	.21	.23	.20	.27
STEP reading score (grade 4)	.20	.18	.28	.25
Physical handicap at 10	.21	.17	.19	.16
Short-term remedial education needs at 10	.11	.10	.20	.15
Long-term remedial education needs at 10	.24	.13	.36	.21
Mental retardation at 10	.05	.18	.02	.06
Learning disability at 10	.07	.15	.43	.37
LMH needs at 10	.14	.30	.65	.35
SMH needs at 10	.04	.11	.51	.26

ous conflicts and high anxiety. The diagnoses of those under mental health care ranged from problems of sexual identity to neurotic symptoms, severe depression, obsessive-compulsive behavior, and paranoid, schizoid behavior.

Among the delinquents were youth (77 males, 26 females) who were or had been involved during adolescence in larceny, burglary, malicious injury, assault and battery, sexual misconduct, and possession and abuse of drugs and also those involved in repeated running away from home, truancy, curfew violations, and unlawful hunting. Excluded were traffic citations and occasional trespassing of property.

PREDICTORS OF SERIOUS MENTAL HEALTH PROBLEMS

Data Available by Age 2. When we combined all the data available to us by age 2, we obtained a multiple R of .37 for the girls and one of .35 for the boys. For both sexes, a low standard of living (at birth or age 2) was the single most powerful predictor of serious mental health problems by age 18, as it had been in the case of the mental health problems diagnosed by age 10. The size of the correlations between early (low) socioeconomic status and later mental health problems was slightly greater for the period between ages 2 and 18 than for the period between 2 and 10 years (r=.31 for SES at age 2 for the girls; r=.21 for standard of living at birth for the boys).

A combination of low SES, congenital defects, and low ratings on physical development by the pediatricians at age 2 was the most effective set of early predictors for the girls (multiple R=.36). A combination of low standard of living and maternal education, moderate to high perinatal stress, difficulty of labor, chronic conditions judged by physicians to lead to minimal brain dysfunction, high activity level and distressing habits of the baby at year 1, and low family stability at age 2 was the most effective set of early predictors for the boys (multiple R=.33).

Ten-Year Data Only. As can be seen from Table 45, correlations between 10-year data and 18-year mental health problems were generally higher than correlations between the earlier data (from birth through age 2) and 18-year outcome. Correlations from year 10 to year 18 also ran higher for boys with serious mental health problems than for girls.

The single most powerful predictor of serious mental health problems by age 18 for the boys was a recognized need for long-term mental health services (six months or more) at age 10. It correlated .65 with the occurrence of serious mental health problems by late adolescence. The correlation rose .76 for boys from homes rated low in socioeconomic status. When we combined the diagnosis of need for mental health services with the presence of a moderate to marked physical handicap and the need for some remedial education at age 10, we obtained a multiple R of .88 for the boys.

Correlations between 10-year data and the occurrence of serious mental health problems in late adolescence among the girls ran somewhat lower, apparently since some of the mental health problems of the teenage mothers (those with illegitimate pregnancies and abortions) had gone unrecognized or had not yet manifested themselves in our 10-year data (see Chapter 8). The single most powerful predictor of serious mental health problems in late adolescence for the girls was a diagnosis of learning disability at age 10 ($r=.37$). Multiple correlations, based on a combination of all 10-year data, rose to $R=.76$. A need for mental health services and the presence of a physical handicap, added to the diagnosis of learning disability at age 10, contributed most of the increased predictive power in the multiple regression equation.

Two-Year and Ten-Year Data Combined. The addition of earlier data (from birth to year 2) to the 10-year data did not improve the multiple correlations for either sex.

IN SUM: A combination of need for long-term mental health services, remedial education, and moderate to marked physical handicap by age 10 was the most powerful predictor of serious mental health problems in late adolescence for the males.

A combination of a learning disability, need for mental health services, and a moderate to marked physical handicap by age 10 was a fairly powerful predictor of serious mental health problems in late adolescence for the females. The predictability of later mental health problems improved considerably from the early to the middle childhood years, indicative of the cumulative effect of biological predisposition and environmental stress during the first 10 years of life. Children from poor homes appeared most vulnerable to this interaction.

PREDICTORS OF DELINQUENCY

Data Available by Age 2. As can be seen in Table 45, correlations between our two-year data and the occurrence of delinquency in adolescence were of about the same magnitude as those between two-year data and mental health problems in late adolescence. They tended to run a little higher for the girls than for the boys and reinforced the impression gleaned from Chapter 8 that girls who became delinquent had more serious behavior problems than boys.

The single most powerful predictor among the early data for the girls was a Cattell IQ score of below 80 ($r=.38$). The correlation between a low Cattell score at age 2 and the occurrence of delinquency in adolescence among girls was higher than any of the correlations from 10-year data to 18-year outcome. (Almost equally powerful for girls from poor homes was the presence of congenital defects: $r=.37$.) When we combined all our data available at age 2, the multiple correlation rose to .44 for the girls, with most of the added predictive power contributed by a low rating of psychological status at age 2 by the psychologist, the presence of distressing habits noted by the mother in infancy, and little maternal education.

The single most powerful predictor among the early data for the boys was a low rating of family stability ($r=.19$). When we combined all our data available by age 2, the multiple correlation rose to .32 for the boys. Low standards of living and maternal education, the presence of congenital defects and a high activity level in the baby, and social immaturity reflected in a low Vineland SQ at age 2 contributed most of the added predictive power.

Ten-Year Data Only. As was the case at age 2, correlations between our 10-year data and the delinquency criterion ran generally higher for the females than the males and improved considerably over the 2–18-year correlations.

The single most powerful predictor of delinquency in late adolescence among girls was the need for long-term mental health services at age 10, with $r=.30$ for all the girls from the 1955 cohort and $r=.32$ for girls from poor homes. Much of the delinquency among the girls was sexual misconduct. When we added our other diagnostic data obtained at age 10 into the multiple regression equation, we obtained a fairly high multiple correlation of .74. A low SES rating at 10, a low PMA IQ and STEP reading score, and a need for remedial education at age 10 were the variables which added most of the additional predictive power to the multiple correlation for the girls.

The most powerful predictors of delinquency in boys were the PMA IQ at age 10 ($r=.24$) and a need for remedial education ($r=.24$). The addition of the other diagnostic data obtained during the 10-year follow-up raised the multiple correlation to $R=.46$, with most of the added predictive power contributed by the presence of a moderate to marked physical handicap, mental retardation, and a low rating of educational stimulation in the home at age 10.

Two-Year and Ten-Year Data Combined. The addition of data available by age 2 to the 10-year variables raised the multiple correlations for both boys and girls, more so for the males than the females. Early variables with added predictive power for the boys were birthweight below 2,500 grams, low social responsiveness at age 1, and both low social maturity and low family stability at age 2.

Early data with added predictive power for the girls were the presence of congenital defects, a Cattell IQ score below 80, and a low rating of psychological (emotional) status by the psychologist at age 2. The added predictive power of these variables helped to account for most of the variance among both male and female delinquents in adolescence.

IN SUM: Predictions of delinquency in adolescence increased from modest correlations at year 2 to high correlations by year 10. Variables that were predictive of delinquency in girls in late adolescence reflected the presence of emotional instability and the need for long-term mental health services in the early elementary grades. Most delinquent boys had learning problems and were in need of long-term remedial education at age 10. Predictions increased if we took into account the family's socioeconomic status (low), maternal education (low), and the presence of physical handicaps at birth or age 10. Predictions were highest when birth, 2-year, and 10-year data were combined.

Key Predictors

In Table 46 we summarize the multiple correlation coefficients and the best single predictors for the various outcomes of this study, using predictors at different points in time. A set of about a dozen

Table 46   Early Predictors of Problems in Childhood and Adolescence: Multiple Correlation Coefficients and Best Single Predictors

Predictors	Males (N=320)	Females (N=313)
*Criteria at Age 2**		
Cattell IQ below 80		
Multiple R	R=.55	R=.59
Congenital defects	r=.43	r=.45
Below normal physical development		
Multiple R	R=.47	R=.37
Congenital defects	r=.26	
Perinatal stress		r=.21
Criteria at Age 10†		
Mental retardation		
Multiple R	R=.57	R=.66
Cattell IQ at 2	r=.46	r=.52
Learning disability		
Multiple R	R=.27	R=.49
Baby's activity level	r=.15	
Cattell IQ		r=.35
Need for LMH services		
Multiple R	R=.36	R=.37
SES at 2	r=.18	
Standard of living at birth		r=.18
Criteria at Age 18†		
Serious mental health problems in adolescence		
Multiple R	R=.35	R=.37
Standard of living at birth	r=.21	
SES at 2		r=.31
Delinquency in adolescence		
Multiple R	R=.32	R=.44
Family stability at 2	r=.19	
Cattell IQ at 2		r=.38
*Criteria at Age 18***		
Serious mental health problems in adolescence		
Multiple R	R=.88	R=.76
LMH child at 10	r=.65	
Learning disability at 10		r=.37
Delinquency in adolescence		
Multiple R	R=.46	R=.74
PMA IQ at 10	r=.24	
LMH child at 10		r=.30

Table 46   (Continued)

Predictors	Males (N=320)	Females (N=313)
Criteria at Age 18‡		
Serious mental health problems in adolescence		
Multiple *R*	*R*=.88	*R*=.60
LMH child at 10	*r*=.65	
Learning disability at 10		*r*=.37
Delinquency in adolescence		
Multiple *R*	*R*=.79	*R*=.81
PMA IQ at 10	*r*=.24	
Cattell IQ at 2		*r*=.38

* Predictions from birth and year 1.

† Predictions from birth, year 1, and year 2.

** Predictions from 10-year data only.

‡ Predictions from birth, year 1, year 2, and 10-year data combined.

variables, some biological, some sociological, and some psychological, appeared with the greatest frequency among the best predictors in our study.

Among the sociological variables were a low level of maternal education (grade 8 or less), a low standard of living, especially at birth but also at ages 2 and 10, and a low rating of family stability.

Among the biological variables were the presence of moderate to severe perinatal stress and the presence of congenital defects at birth and moderate to marked physical handicaps at age 10.

Among the psychological variables were maternal ratings of infant activity level at year 1, a Cattell IQ score below 80 at age 2, a low PMA IQ score (one standard deviation or more) at age 10, and a need for placement in a learning disability class (hyperactive child) or need for six months or more of mental health services by age 10.

Singly or in combination, these variables appeared in all multiple regression equations as key predictors of serious learning and behavior problems in childhood and adolescence. Table 47 shows a comparison of the percentage distribution of these variables among problem children and those in the cohort who did not develop serious learning or behavior problems by age 10 or 18.

We suggest that a screening program addressed to the early identification and prevention of developmental disabilities should

Table 47 Key Predictors of Learning and Behavior Problems in Childhood and Adolescence

Predictor (Birth, Year 2)	Males (N=320) at Age 10				Females (N=313) at Age 10			
	MR (%)	LD (%)	LMH (%)	No Problem (%)	MR (%)	LD (%)	LMH (%)	No Problem (%)
Mother's education: low	46	23	46	15	100	25	40	21
Standard of living at birth: low	92	57	71	41	89	100	82	42
SES at 2: low	62	31	57	23	56	67	57	29
Family stability at 2: low	23	39	14	2	25	38	36	4
Perinatal stress: moderate–severe	15	0	7	12	44	27	27	10
Congenital defects	39	7	0	10	33	11	18	7
Activity level at 1								
Lethargic	18	7	7	0	13	0	0	0
(Very) active	0	69	64	45	0	63	64	47
Cattell IQ below 80 at 2	83	22	25	7	80	100	14	3

Predictor	Males at Age 18				Females at Age 18			
(Birth Years 1, 2, 10)	School Problem (%)	Delinquency (%)	MH Problem (%)	No Problem (%)	School Problem (%)	Delinquency (%)	MH Problem (%)	No Problem (%)
Mother's education: low	25	31	44	14	29	40	20	21
Standard of living at birth: low	61	58	74	41	71	58	66	40
SES at 2: low	26	34	36	23	49	39	65	26
SES at 10: low	76	61	78	46	72	85	83	43
Family stability at 2: low	8	7	14	2	10	15	16	4
Perinatal stress: moderate–severe	8	12	4	12	15	15	13	11
Congenital defects	26	13	9	7	17	27	15	5
Activity level at 1								
Lethargic	8	0	0	0	2	0	0	0
(Very) active	44	53	76	45	51	60	50	47
Cattell IQ below 80 at 2	33	10	14	7	15	33	10	3
Physical handicap at 10: moderate–marked	61	30	29	10	44	13	20	26
Need for LD class at 10	19	7	57	3	21	6	19	4
Need for LMH services at 10	12	8	70	2	14	19	21	1

incorporate information on these variables in their data collection process. We offer them here as tentative signposts to point out potential problem children. We are aware of the need to cross-validate the results of our study of a predominantly Oriental and Polynesian cohort from mostly poor homes with other populations of children representing a wide range of socioeconomic and ethnic groups.

We draw encouragement, however, from the findings of other longitudinal studies with black and white children in the United States and Europe (Great Britain and Denmark). They point to the predictive value of IQ and SES (Anderson et al. 1959; Havighurst et al. 1962; Jones et al. 1971; Kohlberg et al. 1972) and family stability in forecasting later mental health problems. They point also to the enduring effects of perinatal stress on behavior (Mednick and Schulsinger 1969), the importance of infant temperamental traits in behavior disorders (Thomas et al. 1968), and the persistence of problems associated with learning disabilities (Dykman et al. 1973) and acting-out behavior (Robins 1966) in childhood. Recent data from the Collaborative Project in New Orleans with black children (A. C. Smith et al. 1972) and preliminary data from a welfare sample of black, white, and Spanish-speaking children in New York City (Langner 1974) have also shown a dramatic increase in predictive power of psychological assessment if biological and sociological variables are taken into account.

Table 48 shows the cumulative frequencies with which the key predictors appeared among the mentally retarded, those with learning disabilities, the delinquents, and those with serious mental health problems. The presence of four or more of these predictors appears to be a realistic dividing line between most youth at risk for developmental disabilities and most of those who were able to cope with the developmental tasks of childhood and adolescence without developing serious learning and behavior problems.

We are, of course, aware that even our largest correlations between predictor variables and outcomes, though quite significant, do not permit accurate predictions concerning each individual case. What cutting point the practitioner might use to choose *groups* for identification will depend on his or her resources for intervention. As Robins (1966) has pointed out in her

Table 48   Cumulating Early Predictors of Learning and Behavior Disorders

Number of Predictors Present	Criteria					
	MR by 10 (%)	LD by 10 (%)	LMH by 10 (%)	Delinquency by 18 (%)	Mental Health Problems by 18 (%)	No Problems by 10 and 18 (%)
1 or more	100.0	100.0	100.0	100.0	100.0	97.6
2 or more	100.0	100.0	100.0	100.0	100.0	70.6
3 or more	100.0	100.0	92.0	90.0	88.0	49.2
4 or more	100.0	81.0	75.0	72.0	70.0	26.9
5 or more	88.0	54.0	54.0	54.0	50.0	9.1
6 or more	60.0	27.0	37.0	30.0	27.0	2.2
7 or more	44.0	18.0	16.5	16.0	18.0	.6
8 or more	20.0	4.5	4.0	9.0	7.5	0
9 or more	16.0	4.5	4.0	3.0	3.0	0
10 or more	12.0	0	4.0	3.0	3.0	0

study of deviant children, if resources are ample and intervention imposes no distress on children who may not need help, the practitioner may choose to lower the number of predictors required—thus including *all* children at risk for developmental disabilities but also including a proportion of children who would not develop serious learning or behavior problems in childhood or adolescence. If resources are scarce, raising the number of predictors would limit the groups selected to only, but not all, children likely to develop serious learning or behavior disorders. We turn now to the implications of our findings.

CHAPTER 14
Summary and Implications

This study has been concerned with four critical time periods in the lives of youth who were born on the island of Kauai when Hawaii was still a territory and who came of age after the islands had become the fiftieth state of the Union—during two decades of unprecedented ecological, economic, and social change. We were privileged to follow a cohort of more than 600 children and youth from the prenatal period to early and middle childhood and finally to the threshold of adulthood. The sample was a kaleidoscope of ethnic groups—Japanese, Filipino, Hawaiian, Portuguese, Puerto Rican, Chinese, and Anglo-Caucasian—and represented a wide spectrum of socioeconomic classes.

Throughout the two decades of this study, 1955 to 1975, few of the youngsters were lost to our repeated contacts: 96 percent of the 1955 cohort participated in the two-year follow-up, 90 percent in the 10-year follow-up, and 88 percent in the 18-year follow-up. At each phase of this longitudinal study, the parents, their offspring, and professionals from many disciplines and a variety of community agencies gave us their full cooperation. Thus our findings reflect the views of many people who cared enough to share with us their time, their skills, their insights, and their concerns: the parents, the physicians who attended the birth of the children, the public health nurses who followed the mothers through their pregnancies and after delivery and conducted family interviews and home visits when the children were 1 and 10 years old, the pediatricians and psychologists who undertook the developmental screening at age 2 and the diagnostic examinations at age 10, the school personnel who helped us assess the children's academic progress and behavior, the police and probation officers, the social and rehabilitation workers, the public health and mental health professionals and volunteers with whom the troubled ones had contact—and last, but not least, the youth themselves, who gave us their own perspectives on their lives and the effect that significant others had on them as they grew up.

Professional tools varied from behavior observations and screening and diagnostic examinations to interviews and agency records. Professional viewpoints differed, as did our time perspective, as the results of the four phases of the study unfolded. But the independent strands of evidence were tightly interwoven and came together in the end in a pattern that struck us with its cohesiveness and consistency across time.

While our focus has been on those young people who appeared to be most vulnerable to developmental disabilities and serious learning and behavior disorders, we could not help being deeply impressed by the resiliency of the overwhelming majority of children and youth and by their potential for positive change and personal growth. Most young people were competent in coping with their problems, chose their parents as their models, found their family and friends to be supportive and understanding, and expressed a strong continuity with their families in values attached to education, occupational preference, and social expectations.

Our hopefulness was tempered by dismay, however, when we noted the lost opportunities, the stunted growth for the approximately one out of six in this cohort whose lives were "different" and "difficult"—because of early biological impairment, temperamental disposition, the poverty of their homes, the lack of parental education, or family instability. Frequently, many of these factors interacted and exposed them to cumulative biological and psychological stress which was too difficult to cope with unaided.

Summary

The purpose of the follow-up of the children of Kauai in late adolescence was to assess the long-term consequences of learning and behavior disorders identified in early and middle childhood, to discover new problems that arose in adolescence, to evaluate the predictive validity of our earlier assessment tools, to examine the effectiveness of the community's response to youth at risk, and to delineate demographic, family, and interpersonal variables that contributed to improvement. The highlights of our findings follow.

LONG-TERM EFFECTS OF PERINATAL STRESS

Among the 2 percent in this cohort who had suffered *severe* perinatal stress and survived to late adolescence, four out of five had serious behavior, learning, and physical problems. The incidence of mental retardation in this group was ten times, the incidence of serious mental health problems was five times, and the incidence of serious physical handicaps was more than twice that found in the total population of 18-year-olds.

Incidence rates of serious physical handicaps among the 10 percent who had suffered from *moderate* perinatal stress did not differ from the total cohort, but the incidence rate of serious mental health problems was three times as high and that of mental retardation and illegitimate teenage pregnancies was twice as high as that of their peers in the 1955 cohort.

While the physical and, to some extent, the academic and vocational needs of the most severely stressed youth had been attended to by a variety of community agencies, few of the mental health problems among those who suffered from moderate or severe perinatal complications had been recognized.

THE PROGNOSIS FOR LD CHILDREN

About 3 percent of the 1955 cohort had been diagnosed in need of placement in a learning disability class at age 10 on the basis of serious reading and communication problems (in spite of normal intelligence), visual-motor impairment, hyperactivity, and difficulties in attention and concentration. One out of five in this group had physical evidence of "organicity" on pediatric-neurological examinations.

For the overwhelming majority in this group serious problems persisted throughout adolescence: Agency records for four out of five indicated continued academic underachievement confounded by absenteeism, truancy, and a high incidence of repetitive impulsive acting-out behavior that led to problems with the police for the boys, sexual misconduct for the girls, and other mental health problems less often recognized and attended to. Rates of contact with community agencies were nine times as high as that for controls matched by age, sex, socioeconomic status, and ethnicity.

Group tests at age 18 showed continued perceptual-motor problems for most, as well as deficiencies in verbal skills and serious underachievement in reading and writing. Self-reports revealed a pervasive lack of self-assurance and interpersonal competency and a general inadequacy in using their intellectual resources. High external scores on the Locus of Control Scale were indicative of the youths' feeling that their actions were not under their own control.

Educational and vocational plans were nonexistent or unrealistic, and the majority perceived their family, especially their fathers, and their peers as nonsupportive. Professional assistance in adolescence was considered of little help by them. Only one out of four in this group was rated improved by age 18, the lowest proportion among all the groups of youth at risk.

THE PROGNOSIS FOR LMH CHILDREN

About 4 percent of the 1955 cohort had been considered in need of six months or more of mental health services at age 10 because of emotional problems identified by behavior checklists filled out independently by parents and teachers and confirmed by diagnostic evaluations. Four out of five in this group had acting-out problems; the others had been diagnosed as childhood neuroses, schizoid, or sociopathic personalities.

During adolescence more than three out of four in this group had contacts with community agencies, the majority as consequences of persistent serious behavior problems. Rates of contact (many with several agencies) were six times as high as that for controls matched by age, sex, socioeconomic status, and ethnicity. Psychosomatic and psychotic symptoms, sexual misconduct or problems with sexual identity, assault and battery, theft and burglary, drinking and drug abuse, and continued poor academic performance coupled with absenteeism and truancy left these youth few constructive options for the future as they reached young adulthood.

The majority had recognized a need for help, but turned to

their peers for the assistance they did not seek or obtain from their families or community agencies. Only one out of three was judged to have improved by age 18; the improvement rate rose to one out of two among the minority (one out of three) for whom there was some community intervention in adolescence.

THE PROGNOSIS FOR SMH CHILDREN

The prognosis was much more favorable for that group of children (about 10 percent of the 1955 cohort) who, at age 10, had been considered in need of mental health services of less than six months' duration. The overwhelming majority in this group were shy or anxious children who lacked self-confidence and had developed chronic nervous habits to deal with their insecurities.

The overall rate of agency contacts for these youth during adolescence did not differ from that of the total cohort. Only 4 out of 10 had any agency contacts; their problems were less serious and less repetitive than those of the learning disabilities or those considered in need of long-term mental health services at age 10.

Some residual problems persisted in social and achievement behavior at age 18. They were still somewhat socially immature and unwilling to accept responsibility, and they were more handicapped in situations where autonomy and independence were valued.

Only 1 out of 10 had been the beneficiary of intervention by community agencies, but 6 out of 10 were rated improved by age 18. With few exceptions the improved cases had been troubled by a lack of self-confidence, by anxiety, and by chronic nervous habits in childhood. Among the 4 out of 10 who remained unimproved by age 18 were most of the children characterized by high anxiety and acting-out behavior at age 10.

NEW PROBLEMS IN ADOLESCENCE

Most of the youth who became delinquent in adolescence, but only one out of five of the teenage pregnancies, had been considered in need of remedial education, special class placement, or mental health services by age 10. Although these new problems did not differ from controls of the same age and sex on measures of scholastic aptitude and achievement, they expressed a profound lack of faith in the control of their own fate. At age 18 they scored significantly lower than the controls on measures of interpersonal adequacy, maturity, responsiblity, and intellectual efficiency.

Serious problems in social and family life, intense conflict feelings, little self-insight, and low self-esteem were especially characteristic of the pregnant teenagers. Only 1 out of 10 in this group had sought or obtained assistance from community agencies for their pressing mental health needs.

SUBCULTURAL DIFFERENCES

Among all groups of youth at risk in our study, the children of the poor were overrepresented. Among the ethnic groups on the island the Japanese and Chinese were underrepresented; the Filipinos, the Hawaiians, the ethnic mixtures, and, to a slight extent, the Portuguese were overrepresented.

Social class and ethnicity made independent contributions to children's behavior. Social class differences in communication skills (competence in standard English) were greater than ethnic differences and increased during the high school years.

There were significant differences among the three major ethnic groups on the island (Japanese, Filipinos, and Hawaiians and part-Hawaiians) on measures of ascendancy and self-assurance, socialization, and responsiblity. Differences were more pronounced among the girls than the boys. Among the women of Japanese, Filipino, and Hawaiian descent who were scholastically the most successful there were significant differences in life goals, educational and vocational aspirations, and the quality of the relationship with the mother, their main achievement model.

KEY PREDICTORS OF SERIOUS PROBLEMS

About a dozen variables, some biological, some psychological, some sociological, singly and in combination, showed significant relationships across time with poor developmental outcomes at 2 years and serious learning and behavior problems at 10 and 18 years. They were:

1. Moderate to marked degree of perinatal stress
2. Presence of congenital defects
3. Very high or very low levels of infant activity
4. Cattell IQ score below 80 by age 2
5. Low PMA IQ score
6. Moderate to marked degree of physical handicap by age 10

7. Recognized need for placement in a learning disability class by age 10

8. Recognized need for more than six months of mental health services by age 10

9. Low level of maternal education

10. Low standard of living at birth, age 2, or age 10

11. Low family stability at age 2

Predictions of serious learning and behavior problems in childhood and adolescence from data at birth, infancy, and early childhood were consistently higher for children from poor homes and tended to run higher for the girls than for the boys.

SOCIAL AND COMMUNITY INTERVENTION

Overall, only one out of three youths with serious learning and behavior problems in middle childhood and adolescence was the beneficiary of some agency intervention.

There were no socioeconomic differences between youth at risk who did or did not receive the assistance of community agencies on Kauai. The efforts of the various agencies concentrated on those who had the least emotional support in the home, worried the most, and had the greatest conflict feelings. The incidence of intervention varied greatly with the type of problem. There was an *inverse* relationship between the size of the problem group and the proportion of youth who were the beneficiaries of some action by the agencies.

Two out of three among the mentally retarded and nearly half of those with learning disabilities were served by various community agencies during their teens. Four out of ten among the youth considered in need of long-term mental health services at age 10 had the benefit of some intervention by social and community agencies during adolescence. One-third of the new problems in adolescence obtained the assistance of community agencies, but only 1 out of 10 among the youth considered in need of short-term health services at age 10 and only 1 out of 10 among the pregnant teenagers sought or obtained outside help.

Peer friends, parents, and older friends ranked far above *any* kind of professional help as a source of counsel and emotional support. Those considered in need of long-term mental health services turned to peers the most, those with learning disabilities the least. Youth considered in need of long-term mental health services at age 10 regarded outside help given them in adolescence as most effective; youth with learning disabilities regarded outside assistance during their teens as least effective.

FACTORS CONTRIBUTING TO IMPROVEMENT

Overall, less than half of those who did receive some assistance from community agencies during adolescence improved; rates of improvement varied with the type of problem. Although only one out of every four youths with learning disabilities improved in adolescence, one out of three among those who had received some professional help did. And although only one out of three among those considered in need of long-term mental health services by age 10 improved in adolescence, one out of two of those under care did. The highest rate of improvement in adolescence was noted among the youth considered in need of short-term mental health services at age 10: Only 1 out of 10 was provided assistance, but 6 out of 10 improved—with or without the benefit of community intervention.

Significant correlates of improvement were the youths' perception of parental understanding and peer support, a greater belief in the efficacy of their own actions, and their hard work and persistence and better communication skills (competence in standard English).

Socioeconomic status did not affect the improvement rate of youth with learning disabilities and youth considered in need of long-term mental health services at age 10, but it was related to improvement in adolescence among those considered in need of short-term mental health services in childhood. Positive changes in behavior in this group were noted more often for middle-class than lower-class children.

Implications

In summing up the results of the previous phases of this longitudinal study in *The Children of Kauai*, we expressed the hope that our findings might contribute to a better understanding of the quantitative and qualitative aspects of reproductive casualties and the crucial influence of early environment on child development. This hope sustains us as we contemplate the results of our follow-up in late adolescence.

Our prior focus was on those children in our cohort who

suffered from significant developmental disabilities—marked physical handicaps, mental retardation, and serious achievement problems in school. The implications of the findings of the first decade of this study were concerned with prevention and early intervention, the need for multidisciplinary services, training, and research, and the need for setting priorities in the delivery of services to these children.

Our present discussion focuses on significant mental health problems and antisocial behavior in childhood and adolescence. Here we consider the likelihood of their persistence into young adulthood, their biological and temperamental underpinnings, the relationship between social class and vulnerability, and the pervasive effects of early mother-child interaction, perceived locus of control, communication skills, and subcultural differences in socialization. We then turn to a consideration of early developmental screening and different levels of intervention that appear to be called for to meet the pressing mental health needs of children and youth. We close with a consideration of the dilemmas that need to be recognized by legislators, policymakers, and deliverers of services alike, some of which arise out of the potential for conflict between the *individual* rights of parents and children and the increasing *public* concern for the quality of life of the nation's children.

We hope that the results of this study, based on a whole cohort of children in a total community over an extended period of time, will give the reader a perspective that might not be gained from short-term studies with clinic children or selected segments of the population.

THE LIKELIHOOD OF PERSISTENCE

Looking across the spectrum of two decades of development, from the prenatal period to the threshold of adulthood, it appears that many of the childhood learning and behavior disorders that persisted into young adulthood had a strong biological and temperamental underpinning. These should be the prime targets for early intervention. Many of the children recognized in need of placement in a learning disability class or in need of long-term mental health services (six months or more) by age 10 had records of perinatal stress, chronic conditions thought by the physicians attending their birth to be leading to minimal brain dysfunction, congenital defects, and low birthweight. Controls drawn from the same age, sex, socioeconomic status, and ethnic background did not display these factors to a significant extent. In contrast to the learning disability cases and the long-term mental health problems, there were no significant differences between infants later diagnosed in need of short-term mental health care and controls in incidence of perinatal complications, congenital defects, or low birthweight. The majority of these children improved by age 18— with or without the benefit of intervention.

Infant temperamental traits that appeared distressing and nonrewarding to the mother were also noted more frequently, and as early as age 1, among children later recognized as having learning disabilities or needing long-term mental health services whose problems persisted into young adulthood. These temperamental traits may well have been related to biological stress and may have set in motion an early disturbed parent-child relationship that seemed entrenched by age 2, especially in the presence of family instability.

Thoughtful developmental psychologists and clinicians are left to ponder this: Why are there, among the children and youth in this community, as among exceptional individuals whose biographies we read, some who learned to cope, unaided, with great biological and environmental handicaps. Are they anomalies or invincibles who, in the words of poet Lilian Smith, "taught the terrors of their nature and their world to sing"?

In the absence of early biological stress and early family instability, the majority of childhood behavior problems, represented by the children with short-term mental health needs in our cohort, appeared to be temporary, though at the time painful, reactions to environmental stress. Yet the chances for spontaneous improvement in later childhood and adolescence appeared greater for middle-class children than for children of the poor.

SOCIAL CLASS AND VULNERABILITY

We consider it important to keep in perspective that poverty alone was not a sufficient condition for the likelihood of significant coping problems. The overwhelming majority of the control children who were drawn from the same poor and culturally different backgrounds as those with learning disabilities and long-term mental health problems coped very effectively in the second decade of their lives; few of the control children from low and very low SES homes committed any delinquent acts or presented achievement or discipline problems in school.

A low standard of living, especially at birth, increased the likelihood of exposure of the infant to both early biological stress and early family instability. But it was the interaction of early biological stress and early family instability that led to a high risk of developing serious and persistent learning and behavior problems in both lower and middle-class children. Chances for improvement—i.e., changes toward more positive coping skills in adolescence—did not increase with a higher social class position among those with serious learning disabilities and those considered in need of long-term mental health services at age 10.

Our findings, based on the first 18 years of the lives of a multiracial group of children of predominantly Oriental and Polynesian descent, complement those of Robins, who followed "antisocial" white and black children attending public schools into middle age. She noted (1966:304) "That childhood behavior and family patterns rather than class position lead to the hopelessness and alienation found largely in the bottom stratum is further argued by the fact that antisocial children reared in middle-class homes develop into much the same kind of impulsive and imprudent adults that lower-class antisocial children do."

THE HIGH RISK OF TEENAGE MOTHERHOOD

Serious mental health problems were noted in most teenage mothers, a disproportionately larger number of whom had themselves been exposed to moderate perinatal complications as infants. The higher risk of perinatal stress in their offspring can only be inferred from the results of other studies, but the presence of instability in their parents' and their own family and in their relationship with their own infants, documented by their interview responses, makes them a prime target for the perpetuation of a new generation of serious behavior problems and prime candidates for intervention and preventive measures.

EARLY PARENT-CHILD INTERACTION

We were impressed by the pervasive effect of nonrewarding patterns of mother-child interaction which could be documented as early as year 1 by public health nurses who observed in the home and which were verified independently by observations before, during, and after developmental screening examinations at age 2. They were most pronounced in the records of children recognized as having learning disabilities or needing long-term mental health services by age 10 and who developed serious mental health problems or were involved in repeated, serious delinquencies during adolescence.

Often a mother with a relatively low level of education attempted to cope with the needs of an infant she regarded as distressing, nonrewarding, and difficult in an atmosphere of family instability (father absent, home broken, illegitimate birth). By age 2 mother and child were locked in a vicious cycle of increasing frustration for both parent and offspring. By age 10 public health personnel, social workers, and teachers who were unaware of the information obtained on mother-child interaction at ages 1 and 2 noted a pronounced lack of emotional support in the home for most children with serious behavior problems that persisted throughout adolescence. The role of the father appeared more crucial for those with learning disabilities (most of whom were boys) and for the teenage pregnancies. The father's understanding and support or lack of it, his consistent enforcement of rules or lack of it, appeared to play a crucial role in the positive or negative resolution of the developmental problems of his children. Parental attitudes (understanding and support) differentiated significantly between youth with learning and behavior problems who improved in adolescence and those who did not; exposure to different types of intervention by community agencies had a lesser impact.

LOCUS OF CONTROL AND COMPETENCE

We were struck by the pervasive effect of perceived locus of control and competence in communication skills among the youth in this cohort who were at risk for learning disabilities and significant mental health problems. The degree to which youth had faith in the effectiveness of their own actions was related not only to the effectiveness with which they used their intellectual resources in scholastic achievement but also to positive change in behavior in adolescence. An internal locus of control was a significant correlate of improvement. An external locus of control—i.e., a lack of faith in the effectiveness of one's own action—was especially notable among those with serious learning disabilities and the pregnant teenagers, many of whom had serious mental health problems. As a corollary, hard work and persistence were the assets most frequently mentioned by the youth with serious behavior problems in childhood who later improved. Some writers have argued that faith in the control of one's own fate is an illusion. Whatever the validity of this claim, we were impressed that this "illusion" was so effective in the lives of our youth.

Equally pervasive appeared to us the effect of competence in communication skills, i.e., in reading and writing standard English. Limited communication skills led to cumulative problems in coping with cognitive as well as affective demands. Competence in these skills was a major factor contributing to improvement among all the groups of youth at risk.

SUBCULTURAL DIFFERENCES

A recent review of the effectiveness of environmental intervention programs (Horowitz and Paden 1973) noted that most attention in social action programs for children from minority groups has so far focused on the cognitive area, especially on "deficits" or "differences" in concept development and communication skills. The results of our study have made us more cognizant of the lessons taught by the cultural anthropologists—the importance of recognizing and dealing with differences in cultural expectations, parental socialization styles, and the relative strength of affiliative vs. achievement motivation among the different subcultures which make up our pluralistic society.

Among the non-Western subcultures on the island, emphasis on harmony and cooperation, on spontaneity and expressive role behavior, and on personal relationships can easily conflict with demands for competition, individual achievement, and impersonal relationships in the society at large. The majority of our youth coped with the demands of the school system and acquired the cognitive skills valued by the larger society without sacrificing affective ties with their family or ethnic identity. For those with serious learning and behavior disorders, however, intervention programs may well have to address themselves to their need to acquire two cultural response repertoires as well as two languages, issues whose resolution should be facilitated by the passage of the 1974 Bilingual Education Bill. Bicultural and bilingual education creates a need for bridge-builders—models from the subcultures who value their personal and cultural identity as well as competence and excellence. If it succeeds, it should make both teachers and children richer human beings.

DEVELOPMENTAL SCREENING

On the federal and state level, legislative bodies and private advisory boards have recently addressed themselves to the issue of developmental screening. The President's Committee on Mental Retardation (1973) has issued a monograph on the screening and assessment of young children at developmental risk. The 1967 amendments to Title XIX of the Social Security Act, the 1970 Developmental Disabilities Act, and recent state legislation such as California's Child Health and Disability Prevention Program (1974) have recently addressed the issue.

We applaud the quick translation of some of the recommendations made in our previous study into legislative action. Our earlier plea for the importance of screening for developmental disabilities has now been reinforced by our findings related to children with significant mental health problems. Biological stress affecting the central nervous system, temperamental dispositions such as very high or very low levels of infant activity and low social responsiveness, a lag in language or sensorimotor development, excessive dependency and social immaturity, disturbed patterns of mother-child relationships, early family instability—all have been amply documented in the records of those children who later developed serious and persistent behavior problems, including asocial behavior.

Many of these symptoms had been noted and recorded in hospital, birth, and physicians' records or recognized by public health nurses who made home visits in infancy or by the pediatricians and psychologists who conducted the pediatric-psychological screening examinations at age 2; many had also been recognized by the mothers themselves. A behavior checklist filled out independently by the mothers and the teachers and the judicious use of group tests administered in the early elementary grades yielded additional valuable information in middle childhood that red-flagged children at risk for serious learning or behavior problems.

Thus if the periodic developmental screening programs now

contemplated in many American communities are to avoid another avalanche of extensive and repetitive record-keeping, we recommend that they focus on four critical time periods and sources of information:

1. Hospital, birth, and physicians' records containing information about the newborn should be available to community agencies for use and planning with the family for the special needs of the high-risk infant.

2. Developmental screening examinations should be given in the second year of life. They should include information on the physical, sensorimotor, language, and social development of the child and observations on temperamental characteristics and patterns of mother-child interaction. These examinations could be administered by ancillary staff (for instance, nurses) in both public and private settings.

3. Another round of screening in the beginning grades (1 to 3) should be incorporated into the routine school program. It should include a profile of cognitive skills in both the language and nonlanguage area (verbal, reasoning, perceptual, spatial) and a measure of perceptual-motor development, as well as behavior checklists filled out by teachers and parents.

4. A measure of self-concept or locus of control should be filled out by the youth themselves around puberty and might spot the new problems in adolescence.

EARLY INTERVENTION

A recent review by Cowen (1973) on social and community intervention, the first attempt to take stock of this burgeoning field, concluded that prevention and evaluation research are among the weakest links in this new enterprise. In the records of the various community agencies who cooperated with our study and in the interviews with the problem youth in our cohort, we noted that most agency resources still went to corrective and remedial measures for the smallest group of youth at risk, those who were seriously physically handicapped or mentally retarded. Much less attention had been paid to prevention and early intervention, especially among those at risk for serious mental health problems. Only one-third of this group had even been the beneficiaries of remedial or therapeutic measures by community agencies during their teens.

Youth who were doubly vulnerable because of early biological and environmental stress appeared to profit least from intervention after age 10: This was especially true for those with learning disabilities (only one out of three receiving professional help in adolescence improved) and for those considered in need of six months or more of mental health services by age 10 (only one out of two under care improved).

Since many of the key predictors of potential problem behavior were already recognizable by the time of the developmental examinations at age 2, it appears reasonable to suggest that the critical time for intervention for these children should be in early childhood, preferably as early as age 2 and certainly before school entry. The presence of *both* deleterious biological and social factors in the backgrounds of these children will necessitate the diagnostic and healing skills of several disciplines—health and mental health professions, social service agencies, and educators. Successful examples of early intervention with both infants and mothers have recently been reviewed by Horowitz and Paden (1973). The most impressive results have come from programs that began in the second year of life and included individualized day care of the infants and home visits for the purpose of instructing the mother and providing direct stimulation to the infant. The magnitude and maintenance of success appear to be directly correlated with the intensity of the program and the age at which it is begun. We consider it important that parent education include programs that help the parents *first* understand themselves as human beings so that they *then* can become more adequate parents.

The preliminary findings on the effectiveness of early environmental intervention programs raise the issue of a need for a monitoring agent who not only interprets the need for intervention (based on the results of developmental screening examination) to the parents but also sees the family through from infancy to at least the first three grades. Special follow-through kindergartens for children at risk may be another early point of entry for the prevention of serious learning and behavior disorders. The school, in combination with the public health service, could be the prime facilitator for this monitoring system.

During the early grades and especially during latency age, there is need to explore unconventional sources of intervention for problem children: volunteers, retired persons, foster grand-parents, college and high school students who could serve as peer counselors. Examples of imaginative uses of these nonprofes-sionals abound in the Cowen (1973) review of social and com-munity intervention. The interview responses of our troubled youth, especially those in need of long-term mental health ser-vices, suggest that these sources of help have more spontaneous appeal than any kind of professional help, especially during ado-lescence. Emotional support and counsel rendered by such volun-teers are considered at least as effective as intervention by com-munity agencies. Peer counselors and concerned older volunteers could also relieve pressing manpower needs by helping shy, anx-ious, nervous children cope with what appears to be mostly tem-porary distress. This could be done at a lesser emotional cost than if they were left to fend alone. Such volunteers could also be helpful in meeting the pressing mental health needs of pregnant teenagers.

At all social levels and for all types of learning and behavior problems, there is need to involve *both* parents in any kind of in-tervention program since their understanding of the needs of the troubled child and their emotional support appear to play a cru-cial role in the likelihood of positive change to better coping skills.

Whether or not parents or youth will avail themselves of these different levels of intervention may ultimately depend on the congruency of expectations and efforts by the deliverers and recip-ients of the services. Without it new programs (or more commonly old programs with new names), more professional man-power, more use of paraprofessionals or nonprofessionals, and even more financial support for the needs of children will not spell suc-cess in intervention.

It has been troublesome to us to notice that during five de-cades of concern with the mental health needs of the nation's chil-dren, the different types of intervention programs tried—the child guidance approach, the community mental health approach, the systems approach, and now community and social intervention—appear to reach the same magic number: only *one out of three* of those in need. Could it be that there is, in Daniel P. Moynihan's words, "a maximum feasible misunderstanding" between the well-meaning efforts of concerned legislators, policymakers, and deliverers of social services and the real needs of two-thirds of potential clients? We do not know; but that number *ought* to be a cause for concern, a continued concern with the evaluation of the effectiveness of new and unconventional intervention programs.

SOME DILEMMAS OF INTERVENTION

Throughout this book we have focused on the early identification of high-risk youth and the value of preventive rather than remedial or therapeutic measures. Our commitment, we trust, is being shared by an increasing number of people who shape social policy and who care for the needs of individual children. Those concerned with prevention and early intervention may, however, have to face up to and live with a dilemma that arises out of the possibility of conflict between the increasing *public* concern for the quality of life of America's children and the increasing awareness of the *individual* rights of parents and children.

The dilemmas of intervention are somewhat reminiscent of Tevye's dialogue in *Fiddler on the Roof*. And, like him, we may have to maintain a precarious balance—and a sense of humor—when we advocate intervention in the lives of children and their families, either enrichment when it is applied as a preventive measure or remediation when it is corrective.

On the one hand, there is increasing concern for the *needs* of children and youth that is reflected in social policy and new legislation dealing with prevention and early intervention. On the other hand, there is an increasing awareness of the *rights* of children and parents—for instance, the access to diagnostic information, the right of privacy, the rights of the mentally handicapped, the class action suits by parent groups against "labeling" and "tracking"—in other words, the right to say no to public intervention, no matter how well-meaning.

On the one hand, there is more emphasis on earlier and extensive screening for all types of developmental disabilities, including childhood learning and behavior disorders, with the implicit assumption that once children at risk are identified and their parents or guardians are informed, they will be "taken care of." On the other hand, there are the limitations of existing community agencies in handling present case loads, even before the increase that is to be expected when routine screening reaches all children eligible for medical assistance or all children under six.

On the one hand, there is greater stress on massive public intervention and extensive use of a variety of professionals, para-professionals, and nonprofessionals in the community. On the other hand, there is the reality that most children and youth in trouble appear to turn to family and peers for help, not to outside sources.

On the one hand, there is greater awareness of the increasing risks of biological and psychosocial stress among the children of the poor. On the other hand, there is the persistent inability of public agencies to reach those among the poor who are the most at risk.

On the one hand, there are increasing demands for complex problem-solving, communication, and coping skills needed for *all* our youth to survive in a technological society exposed to rapidly accelerating change. On the other hand, there is the desire by a substantial number of minorities to preserve or recapture a cultural identity of their own in a pluralistic nation.

The resolution of the conflicting demands between the individual rights of parents and children and the public and private responsibility to take care of their needs may be facilitated by federal or state legislation, by greater expenditure of money from the public and private sector, by more investment in manpower training, and by translation of research findings into social action programs. But in the end, an effective balance cannot be reached unless people of goodwill among all parties concerned, the helping agencies, the parents, and the youth themselves, join in a common cause and reach a consensus on their mutual expectations. And an effective balance *must* be sought, for, in the words of Erik Erikson:

> The most deadly of all possible sins is the mutilation of a child's spirit.

APPENDIXES

APPENDIX 1
Summary of Major Findings from Perinatal Period to Age 10

Reproductive and Environmental Casualties

1. Of pregnancies reaching four weeks' gestation, an estimated 237 per 1,000 ended in loss of the conceptus. The rate of loss formed a decreasing curve from a high of 108 per 1,000 women under observation in the period 4–7 weeks of gestation to a low of 3 in the period 32–35 weeks.

2. Neonatal, infant, and childhood mortality rates on Kauai were all very low, reflecting a near minimum number of unfavorable postnatal influences. The perinatal mortality rate based on fetal deaths of 20 weeks and more and on infant deaths under 28 days was 35.9 per 1,000 pregnancies. The number of reported fetal deaths of 20 or more weeks was almost twice the number of deaths during the first month after birth. There were 11.7 first-week deaths per 1,000 live births and 13.8 deaths under 28 days.

3. The liveborn were classified as to presence and severity of physical and mental handicapping conditions of perinatal origin, and estimates were made of the type of care required. In the first two years of life, minor perinatal handicaps had been recognized in 7 percent of the liveborn in the time sample: 6.3 percent had conditions requiring short-term medical and nursing services, largely prematurity care, and physical defects requiring surgery

and other specialized care; 3.7 percent were severely handicapped and required long-term medical, special educational, or custodial services. This last group included children with severe physical defects, children with combined physical defects and mental retardation, and a group of mentally retarded children without recognizable physical defects by age 2.

4. By age 10, 6.6 percent of the children in the time sample were moderately or severely physically handicapped as a result of physical or mental defects or both. Included were 2.3 percent in classes for the mentally retarded. Ten percent of the children were in grades below their chronological age. Forty percent received grades of D or worse in one or several basic skill subjects. In each subject more than one-fourth of all children had grades of D and about 5 percent were failing. About one-fourth had some behavior problems.

5. Among services needed for these children by age 10, by far the greatest demand was for remedial help in the basic skill subjects. Twenty-one percent of the children were in need of long-term and 18 percent of short-term help. Over five times as many children required special educational services (39 percent) as those who required special medical care, and almost twice as many had emotional problems interfering with school progress (13 percent). The greatest need of these 10-year-olds—required by almost one-third of them—was for long-term educational or mental health services or both.

6. In sum, for each 1,000 live births on Kauai there were an estimated 1,311 pregnancies that had advanced to four weeks' gestation, 186 having ended in fetal deaths before 20 weeks' gestation and 25 more between 20 weeks and term. The 1,000 live births yielded an estimated 844 surviving children at age 2 who were free of any observed physical defect requiring special care and who had IQs of at least 85. By age 10, only 660 of these children were functioning adequately in school and had no recognized physical, intellectual, or behavior problem.

Birthweight and Gestational Differences

1. While the overall incidence of low birthweight (2,500 grams or less) was 7.4 percent, it was estimated that 3.2 percent were the *small, normal* babies of small mothers (because of the

characteristics of our study population, this proportion is probably higher than it would be in many mainland communities); 2.6 percent were gestationally *premature* (less than 37 weeks' gestation); and 1.6 percent were *dysmature*.

2. The proportion of infants with birthweight of 2,500 grams or less, both less than 37 weeks' gestation and 37 weeks or more, was highest for mothers (*a*) with a history of giving birth to small infants, (*b*) who gained less than 10 pounds during pregnancy, (*c*) were of short stature, and (*d*) were unmarried. A history of previous fetal deaths increased the chance of giving birth to small, preterm infants, and a low prepregnancy weight was associated with small babies born at term (dysmatures). The percentages were highest for mothers in the lowest socioeconomic group for most variables.

3. Except for the very few babies (less than 1 percent) weighing less than 1,500 grams at birth, the much larger group weighing 1,500 to 2,500 grams had approximately the same proportion of intellectual, emotional, and physical problems as their peers who had been born heavier; only for perceptual problems did they have a significant excess.

Ethnic Differences

1. Infant mortality rates dropped sharply among the two largest immigrant groups to Kauai, the Japanese and the Filipinos; the Hawaiian population showed a lesser rate of improvement.

2. When social class was held constant, there remained significant differences in abilities and achievement among children from the five ethnic groups on Kauai at ages 2 and 10. Significant differences were also found in the language styles and amount of educational stimulation transmitted by their families. Children of Filipino, Hawaiian, and Portuguese descent had lower mean scores on the Cattell and PMA tests and more achievement and behavior problems than did Anglo-Caucasian and Japanese children.

Sex Differences

1. A difference between the sexes in the rate of intellectual maturation favored the girls from ages 2 to 10, resulting in higher correlations between their IQs and measures of parental ability than for the boys.

2. Girls appeared to be more responsive than boys to achievement demands made by the family. The difference between the sexes in favor of the girls was significant for all environmental ratings, especially educational stimulation.

Predictive Value of Early Examinations

1. The diagnoses for children with significant handicaps—physical, mental, or both—by age 2 were largely confirmed at age 10.

2. The poorest rate of prediction among the physical health problems involved children with eye defects. Only half of those identified as having strabismus at age 2 had had any eye problem diagnosed by age 10. An equal number of additional eye problems had been diagnosed by that time, some severe enough to affect school progress. Some might have been prevented by earlier diagnosis with special sensory screening procedures.

3. The best single predictor of IQ and achievement at age 10 was the Cattell IQ score at age 2. A combination of Cattell IQ, pediatricians' rating, Vineland SQ, perinatal stress score, and parental SES yielded a moderately high positive correlation ($R=.58$) with 10-year IQ; most of the added predictive power was contributed by parental SES. For children with IQs below 80 at age 2, a combination of Cattell IQ and pediatricians' rating of intelligence yielded a high positive correlation ($R=.80$) with the IQ score at 10 years.

4. A combination of deprived environment and retarded intellectual development noted by pediatricians and psychologists for children before age 2 more accurately predicted later serious achievement problems in school than did either the examinations or environmental ratings alone.

APPENDIX 2
Perinatal Stress Scores

Mild (Score 1)	Moderate (Score 2)
Mild: preeclampsia, essential hypertension, renal insufficiency or anemia; controlled diabetes or hypothyroidism; positive Wasserman and no treatment; acute genito-urinary infection third trimester; untreated pelvic tumor producing dystocia; treated asthma	Marked: preeclampsia, essential hypertension, renal insufficiency or anemia; diabetes under poor control; decompensated cardiovascular disease requiring treatment; untreated thyroid dysfunction; confirmed rubella first trimester; nonobstetrical surgery: general anesthesia, abdominal incision or hypotension
Vaginal bleeding second or third trimester; placental infarct; marginal placenta previa; premature rupture of membranes; amnionitis; abnormal fetal heart rate; meconium-stained amniotic fluid (exclude if breech); confirmed polyhydramnios	Vaginal bleeding with cramping; central placenta previa; partial placenta abruptio; placental or cord anomalies
Rapid, forceful, or prolonged un-productive labor; frank breech or persistent occiput posterior; twins; elective cesarean section; low for-ceps with complications; cord pro-lapsed or twisted and oxygen administered to newborn	Chin, face, brow, or footling presen-tation; emergency cesarean section; manual or forceps rotation, midforceps or high forceps or breech and oxygen administered under 5 minutes
Breathing delayed 1–3 minutes; inter-mittent central cyanosis and oxygen administered under 1 minute; cry weak or abnormal; bradycardia	Breathing delayed 3–5 minutes; gasping; intermittent central cyanosis and oxygen administered over 1 minute; cry delayed 5–15 minutes
Birth injury excluding central nervous system; jaundice; hemorrhagic disease mild; pneumonia, rate of respiration under 40 and oxygen administered intermittently; birth weight 1,800–2,500 grams and oxygen administered intermittently or incubator or other special care; oral antibiotic to newborn; abnormal tone or Moro reflex; irritability	Major birth injury and temporary central nervous system involvement; spasms; pneumonia, rate of respiration over 40 and oxygen administered intermittently; apnea and oxygen administered inter-mittently or resuscitation under 5 minutes; birthweight 1,800–2,500 grams, fair suck and oxygen administered or incubator; antibiotics administered intravenously; cry absent

Severe (Score 3)

Eclampsia; renal or diabetic
coma; treated pelvic tumor

Complete placenta abruptio;
congenital syphilis of the
newborn

Transverse lie; emergency cesarean
section; manual rotation, midforceps
or high forceps or breech extraction
and oxygen administered 5 minutes
or more

Breathing delayed over 5 minutes;
no respiratory effort; persistent
cyanosis and oxygen administered
continuously; cry delayed over
15 minutes

Major birth injury and persistent
central nervous system involvement;
exchange transfusion; seizure;
hyaline membrane disease; pneumonia,
rate of respiration over 60 and
oxygen administered continuously,
resuscitation over 5 minutes;
birthweight under 1,800 grams
and oxygen administered or
special feeding; meningitis;
absent Moro reflex

APPENDIX 3
Case Summaries of LD, LMH, and SMH Children

LD Children

Female. Perinatal stress: 0. SES: low. Emotional support and educational stimulation in home: low.

Active, affectionate infant but anxious, fearful, slow two-year-old. Mother easygoing, indifferent. Cattell IQ 81; Vineland SQ 105. *At age 10*: WISC verbal IQ 72, performance IQ 87, full-scale IQ 77; Bender-Gestalt score 2. Perceptual problems. Repeated one grade but receiving D's and F's. *During adolescence*: Chronic school nonattendance. Counseling (no improvement noted). STEP scores lowest 5th percentile. Financial aid from Social Services. *Interview ratings at age 18*: Poor attitudes toward school, lack of realistic future plans, little goal and value differentiation. Rejecting parents; poor family and social adjustment. Very great conflict feelings, very low self-esteem. *Rated unimproved*.

Male. Perinatal stress: 0. SES: low. Emotional support: high. Educational stimulation: average.

Considered fairly active infant; temper tantrums. Ambivalent, fearful, suspicious, hesitant two-year-old. Mother good-humored, affectionate, calm with infant, but at two years indifferent, distant, matter-of-fact. Cattell IQ 107; Vineland SQ

133. *At age 10*: WISC verbal IQ 95, performance IQ 85, full-scale IQ 89; Bender-Gestalt score 4. PMA Spatial Factor 56, Perceptual Factor 59. D's in writing and arithmetic. Described as impulsive, has unusual fears, poor motor coordination, restless. *During adolescence*: SCAT and STEP scores lowest 5th percentile except STEP math (24th percentile); Bender-Gestalt score 1. *Interview ratings at age 18*: Favorable attitude toward school but content to get by; realistic future plans; family relationships and identifications strong. Absence of conflict feelings, fair self-esteem, but little goal and value differentiation. *Rated improved.*

Female. Perinatal stress: 1. SES: very low. Emotional support and educational stimulation in home: very low.

Very active, cuddly infant but throws self on floor. Active, friendly, independent, restless two-year-old. Mother easygoing, careless, erratic, punitive. Cattell IQ 87; Vineland SQ 104. *At age 10*: WISC verbal IQ 82, performance IQ 85, full-scale IQ 82; Bender-Gestalt score 1; PMA Perceptual Factor 76. Repeated one grade and receiving D's and F's. Described as quarrelsome, negativistic, distractible, restless; lying and tantrums. *During adolescence*: Overweight, asthmatic; school referrals for drinking and smoking; other physical problems. SCAT and STEP scores lowest 15th percentile; Bender-Gestalt score 5. Frequent school absences. *Interview ratings at age 18*: Favorable attitude toward school but realism of future plans ambiguous. In conflict with mother, strong identification with father, family adjustment fair. Goal and value differentiation and self-insight high. Self-esteem fair, conflict feelings noted. *Rated unimproved.*

Female. Perinatal stress: 1. SES: very low. Emotional support and educational stimulation in home: low.

Fairly active, cuddly, affectionate infant. Mother unemotional, reserved, withdrawn, childlike. *At age 10*: WISC verbal IQ 87, performance IQ 80, full-scale IQ 83; Bender-Gestalt score 4. Perceptual problem noted. D's and F's in reading and arithmetic. Described as restless, distractible, unable to concentrate, lacking self-confidence, shy. *During adolescence*: Police report of shoplifting. Pregnant and married at 17. SCAT and STEP scores lowest 7th percentile; Bender-Gestalt score 2. *Interview ratings at age*

18: Favorable attitude toward school but content just to get by. Family adjustment and identifications adequate. Little self-insight, fair self-esteem. Goal and value differentiation limited, few conflict feelings. *Rated unimproved.*

Female. Perinatal stress: 1. SES: low. Educational stimulation in home: low. Emotional support: average.

Cuddly, fairly active infant; temper tantrums. Anxious, bashful, uncommunicative two-year-old. Mother intelligent, good-humored, responsible, reasonably relaxed, kind. Vineland SQ 107. *At age 10*: WISC performance IQ 93, verbal IQ 74, full-scale IQ 81; Bender-Gestalt score 1. D's and F's in reading, writing, arithmetic. Described as unpopular, teased, stubborn; bites nails, feelings easily hurt. *During adolescence*: School counselor notes slow, infantile behavior; overweight. SCAT and STEP scores lowest 5th percentile except STEP math (28th percentile). *Interview ratings at age 18*: Favorable attitude toward school but content to get by, future plans ambiguous in realism. Social life poor, but family adjustment and identifications adequate. Very intense conflict feelings, some goal and value differentiation, little self-insight, low self-esteem. *Rated unimproved.*

Male. Perinatal stress: 2. SES: middle class. Educational stimulation: average. Emotional support: high.

At age 10: WISC verbal IQ 85, performance IQ 82, full-scale IQ 82; Bender-Gestalt score 10. Severe problems in motor coordination. Hyperactive, distractible, immature, short interest span, lisps. D's in reading, writing, arithmetic. Growth retardation. *During adolescence*: SCAT and STEP scores 15th to 38th percentile; Bender-Gestalt score 6. *Interview ratings at age 18*: Very favorable attitude toward school, high achievement motivation, very realistic future plans. Family adjustment and identifications good. High self-insight and self-esteem, great degree of goal and value differentiation. *Rated improved.*

Male. Perinatal stress: 1. SES: very low. Educational stimulation and emotional support in home: low.

Fairly active, cuddly infant; bashful, dependent, solemn two-year-old. Mother responsible, energetic, takes things in stride, matter-of-fact, kind. Cattell IQ 79; Vineland SQ 93. *At age 10*:

WISC full-scale IQ 80, verbal IQ 72, performance IQ 92; Bender-Gestalt score 1. Difficulties in concentration and attention; is stubborn, lies. Grades F's. *During adolescence*: Known to police for burglary and malicious injury. Low school performance with referral to Learning Center. SCAT and STEP scores lowest 15th percentile. *Interview ratings at age 18*: Favorable attitude toward school, content to get by, future plans somewhat unrealistic. Family adjustment and identifications adequate. Little self-insight and goal and value differentiation. Self-esteem fair. *Rated unimproved*.

Male. Perinatal stress: 0. SES: low. Educational stimulation: average. Emotional support: low.

Fairly active, cuddly infant; bashful, slow, uncommunicative two-year-old. Mother intelligent, stable, responsible, reasonably relaxed, kind, affectionate. Vineland SQ 109. *At age 10*: WISC full-scale IQ 74, verbal IQ 62, performance IQ 92; Bender-Gestalt score 4. Memory difficulties, letter reversals; easily distracted, restless, anxious. Repeated one grade; 10-year grades D's and F's. *During early adolescence*: Known to Public Health Nursing; later contact with school counselor because of poor effort. SCAT and STEP scores lowest 25th percentile; Bender-Gestalt score 2. *Interview ratings at age 18*: Attitude toward school favorable, content to get by, future plans somewhat unrealistic. Family adjustment fair, father rejecting, identifies with mother, strong feeling of security. Little conflict, no self-insight or goal and value differentiation, low self-esteem. *Rated unimproved*.

Male. Perinatal stress: 0. SES: low. Educational stimulation: low. Emotional support: average.

Very active, cuddly infant; active, dependent, restless, nervous, distractible two-year-old. Mother calm, self-confident, takes things in stride, restrictive. Cattell IQ 90; Vineland SQ 110. *At age 10*: WISC verbal IQ 94, performance IQ 92, full-scale IQ 92; significant subtest scatter and reversals; Bender-Gestalt score 2. Distractible, tantrums, restless, impulsive. D's and F's in reading, writing, arithmetic. *During adolescence*: Known to police for minor theft; remedial program in school. SCAT and STEP scores lowest 15th percentile. *Interview ratings at age 18*: Mixed reactions to school, realistic future plans. Strong identification with mother, father rejecting. Overall family adjustment good. High degree of self-insight, extent of goal and value differentiation great, some conflict. Quite high self-esteem. *Rated improved.*

Male. Perinatal stress: 0. SES: low. Educational stimulation and emotional support in home: low.

Very active, cuddly infant; agreeable, alert, serious, persevering two-year-old. Mother intelligent, stable, affectionate, takes things in stride. Cattell IQ 104; Vineland SQ 109. *At age 10*: WISC verbal IQ 100, performance IQ 96, full-scale IQ 98; Bender-Gestalt score 1. Repeated a grade and attaining D's and F's in reading and writing. *During adolescence*: SCAT and STEP scores lower third except quantitative scores (49th percentile). Articulation problem; police contact. *Interview ratings at age 18*: Favorable attitude toward school but content to get by. Family adjustment and identifications fair. Little conflict, little self-insight. Some goal and value differentiation. Self-esteem fair. *Rated unimproved.*

Female. Perinatal stress: 2. SES: low. Educational stimulation: low. Emotional support: very low.

At age 10: WISC full-scale IQ 77, verbal IQ 70, performance IQ 90; Bender-Gestalt score 6. Concentration and attention difficulties; irritable, negativistic; lies and steals. Grades D's and F's. *During adolescence*: Referred to Mental Health for behavior problems in school; recommendation for long-range psychiatric treatment for mother and child, but treatment plan not followed. Withdrew from school at age 15½. Refused interview but indicated via questionnaire that she was out on own, school of no importance, family relationships poor. Regarded self as confused. *Rated unimproved.*

Male. Perinatal stress: 0. SES: low. Educational stimulation: average. Emotional support: high.

Bashful and solemn two-year-old. Mother easygoing, affectionate, takes things in stride. Cattell IQ 95; Vineland SQ 110. *At age 10*: WISC verbal IQ 79, performance IQ 75, full-scale IQ 75; Bender-Gestalt score 8. Grades D's and F's. Lacks self-confidence, bites nails. *During adolescence*: SCAT and STEP scores lowest 10th percentile except STEP math (17th percentile). Minor police contact for trespassing. Refused interview. Questionnaire revealed no future plans beyond high school graduation; regarded self as undecided and confused. Many worries, family relationships satisfactory. *Rated unimproved.*

Male. Perinatal stress: 0. SES: very low. Educational stimulation and emotional support in home: very low.

Quiet infant; awkward, slow two-year-old. Mother indulgent, affectionate, worrisome, kind. Cattell IQ 86; Vineland SQ 90. *At age 10*: WISC verbal IQ 79, performance IQ 93, full-scale IQ 84; Bender-Gestalt score 6. Impaired perceptual-motor functioning. Distractible, negativistic, bullying, restless, destructive. Pediatric exam notes subtle neurological abnormalities. Grades D's and F's. *During adolescence*: School reports continued limited functioning, social work contacts with parents. SCAT and STEP scores lowest 23rd percentile. *Interview ratings at age 18*: Low achievement motivation, mixed feelings toward school, realistic future vocational plans, strong family support and identifications. Much conflict, little self-insight, no goal and value differentiation. Self-esteem very low. *Rated unimproved.*

Male. Perinatal stress: 0. SES: very low. Educational stimulation and emotional support in home: low.

Active infant, keeps to self, head-banging. Slow, solemn, tense, uncommunicative two-year-old. Mother affectionate, worried, good-humored, kind. Vineland SQ 67. *At age 10*: WISC full-scale IQ 82, verbal IQ 87, performance IQ 79; Bender-Gestalt score 2. Visual-motor problem. Repeated one grade. Grades D's and F's in reading, writing, arithmetic. Asthmatic, shy, feelings easily hurt. *During adolescence*: SCAT and STEP scores lowest 15 percentile. *Interview ratings at age 18*: Favorable attitude toward school, future plans fairly realistic. Family adjustment and support adequate. Some self-insight, conflict feelings, goal and value differentiation great. Fair self-esteem. *Rated improved.*

Male. Perinatal stress: 0. SES: low. Educational stimulation: low. Emotional support: average.

Fairly active, cuddly infant; distractible, passive, restless two-year-old. Mother responsible, outgoing, affectionate, kind, mature. Cattell IQ 95; Vineland SQ 124. *At age 10*: WISC full-scale IQ 99, verbal IQ 96, performance IQ 103; Bender-Gestalt score 7. Definite perceptual problem. Unusual fears. Repeated one school year. Grades D's and F's. *During adolescence*: SCAT and STEP scores lower 35th percentile. *Interview ratings at age 18*: Favorable attitude toward school, content to get by. Very realistic future plans. Good family adjustment, strong feelings of security. Little evidence of conflict, some goal and value differentiation and self-insight. Fair self-esteem. *Rated improved*.

Female. Perinatal stress: 0. SES: middle class. Educational stimulation and emotional support in home: low.

Fairly active, cuddly, affectionate infant; deliberate, slow two-year-old. Mother indulgent, warmhearted, affectionate, easily angered. Cattell IQ 86; Vineland SQ 124. *At age 10*: WISC verbal IQ 79, performance IQ 94, full-scale IQ 85; Bender-Gestalt score 6. Grades D's and F's. Passive, immature, lacks confidence; temper tantrums. *During adolescence*: SCAT and STEP scores lowest 25th percentile. *Interview ratings at age 18*: Content to get by in school, attitude toward school and future plans mixed. Very poor social life. Insecure in family relationships. Little self-insight, little goal and value differentiation. Great conflict feelings, very low self-esteem. *Rated unimproved*.

Male. Perinatal stress: 0. SES: low. Educational stimulation and emotional support in home: average.

Very active, cuddly infant; agreeable, serious two-year-old. Mother intelligent, easygoing, kind, and at two years careless. Cattell IQ 113; Vineland SQ 109. *At age 10*: WISC verbal IQ 110, performance IQ 97, full-scale IQ 104; Bender-Gestalt score 3. Grades D's and F's. Attention and concentration difficulties, restless, quarrels easily, irritable. *During adolescence*: SCAT and STEP scores 20th to 55th percentile. *Interview ratings at age 18*: Mixed reactions toward school, content to get by. Future plans not very realistic. Family adjustment poor, parents rejecting. No self-insight, no goal and value differentiation, some conflict. Self-esteem very low. *Rated unimproved*.

Male. Perinatal stress: 0. SES: low.

Fairly active, cuddly infant; head-banging. Agreeable, solemn two-year-old. Mother indulgent, suggestible, erratic, discontent, worrisome; at two years, kind and takes things in stride. *At age 10*: WISC verbal IQ 81, performance IQ 74, full-scale IQ 75; Bender-Gestalt score 8. Depressed, tantrums. Repeated grade in school. Grades D's and F's. *During adolescence*: Bender-Gestalt score 4. Public Health Nursing contact for one year. *Interview ratings at age 18*: Favorable school attitude, high motivation, future plans mixed regarding realism. Good family adjustment, strong identifications. Great goal and value differentiation, some conflict, some self-insight. Self-esteem fair. *Rated improved.*

Female. Perinatal stress: 0. SES: very low. Educational stimulation and emotional support in home: very low.

Very active, cuddly infant; head-banging. Hostile, restless, stubborn, suspicious two-year-old. Mother affectionate, good-humored, reasonably relaxed with infant, but considered indifferent and childlike with two-year-old. Cattell IQ 74; Vineland SQ 121. *At age 10*: WISC full-scale IQ 70, verbal IQ 82, performance IQ 62; significant perceptual impairment; Bender-Gestalt score 8. Repeated a year in school. Grades D's and F's in reading, writing, arithmetic. Distractible, stubborn, feelings easily hurt. *During adolescence*: Known to Special Services, Mental Health, police, Family Court. SCAT and STEP scores 11th to 85th percentile; Bender-Gestalt score 4. *Interview ratings at age 18*: Mixed reactions toward school, content to get by. Very poor family adjustment, feelings of security weak, very rejecting father. Little self-insight, no goals and value differentiation, some conflict. Very low self-esteem. *Rated unimproved.*

Three additional LD children (two with perinatal stress scores of 0, one with a perinatal stress score of 1) had incomplete follow-up data.

LMH Children

Female. Perinatal stress: 1. SES: low. Educational stimulation: low. Emotional support: very low.

Very active infant, "troublemaker"; aggressive, restless, independent two-year-old. Mother relaxed, easygoing, matter-of-fact, reasonable, takes things in stride. Cattell IQ 91; Vineland SQ 122. *At age 10*: PMA IQ 106; Bender-Gestalt score 6. Distractible, irritable; temper tantrums, bullying; depressed, negativistic toward mother, abused by father. Living with relatives, involved in truancy and delinquent behavior. School achievement satisfactory. *During adolescence*: Active with Special Services, Mental Health. Psychiatrist's diagnosis: hysterical personality disorder. Frequent runaways and pregnant at 17 and again at 18 years. Heavily involved in drugs. Dropped out of school but had returned to special adult continuation program at time of interview. *Interview ratings at age 18*: Very favorable attitude toward school, realistic vocational plans. Family adjustment poor, very rejecting father, but strong mother-daughter relationship. Some goal and value differentiation, great feelings of conflict, high degree of self-insight. Self-esteem fair. *Rated unimproved.*

Female. Perinatal stress: 1. SES: very low. Educational stimulation and emotional support in home: low.

Fairly active infant; keeps to self; head-banging. Bashful, fearful, indecisive, slow, quiet two-year-old. Mother stable, mature, happy, affectionate, self-confident, takes things in stride. Cattell IQ 91; Vineland SQ 95. *At age 10*: WISC full-scale IQ 89, verbal IQ 71, performance IQ 111. Anxious, withdrawn, lacks self-confidence. Schizoid functioning with poor integration of affect and evidence of poor judgment and lack of contact with reality. Family problems noted by age 10. *During adolescence*: School noted frequent cutting classes. SCAT and STEP scores lower 3rd percentile. *Interview ratings at age 18*: Mixed reactions toward school, content to get by, future plans unrealistic. Family adjustment fair, relationships with parents satisfactory. No goal and value differentiation, intense conflict feelings, little self-insight. Self-esteem fair. *Rated unimproved.*

Male. Perinatal stress: 0. SES: very low. Educational stimulation: low. Emotional support: very low.

Agreeable, independent, restless two-year-old. Mother matter-of-fact, takes things in stride. Cattell IQ 90; Vineland SQ 110. *At age 10*: WISC verbal IQ 94, performance IQ 118, full-scale IQ 106; Bender-Gestalt score 2. Grades D's and F's in reading, writing, arithmetic. Wets bed; temper tantrums; fearful, shy. Psychologist notes poor self-image, aggressive impulse life, problems in relationship with parents. *During adolescence*: Diagnostic evaluation by Mental Health followed by Social Services. Police contact for minor burglary episode. SCAT and STEP scores 3rd to 37th percentile. *Interview ratings at age 18*: Favorable attitude toward school. Realistic future plans. Parental relationships satisfactory, overall feelings of security and family adjustment good. Little goal and value differentiation, few feelings of conflict, little insight. Self-esteem fair. *Rated improved.*

Male. Perinatal stress: 0. SES: low. Educational stimulation and emotional support in home: low.

Very active infant; agreeable, independent, sociable two-year-old. Mother responsible, patient, kind, energetic. Cattell IQ 100; Vineland SQ 104. *At age 10*: WISC full-scale IQ 91, verbal IQ 76, performance IQ 108; Bender-Gestalt score 0. D's and F's in school. Severely asthmatic. Depressed, anxious, fearful. *During adolescence*: Active with Social Services. Foster home placement (one year). SCAT and STEP scores 11th to 42nd percentile. *Interview ratings at age 18*: Mixed reactions toward school, achievement motivation fair, future plans fairly realistic. Family adjustment good, strong feelings of security and identifications. Goal and value differentiation great. Some conflict feelings, some self-insight. Self-esteem fair. *Rated improved.*

Male. Perinatal stress: 1. SES: low. Educational stimulation and emotional suport in home: low.

Fairly active, affectionate infant; active, eager, responsive, independent, restless two-year-old. Mother good-humored, matter-of-fact, indulgent, resourceful. Cattell IQ 113; Vineland SQ 133. *At age 10*: WISC verbal IQ 101, performance IQ 97, full-scale IQ 99; Bender-Gestalt score 3. Stutters, blinks, lacks confidence; restless, inability to concentrate. Psychologist notes considerable tension, anxiety, emotional insecurity. *During early adolescence*: Mental Health for drug therapy and individual psychotherapy; failed to keep appointments. SCAT and STEP scores 6th to 33rd percentile. *Interview ratings at age 18*: Very favorable attitude toward school, high achievement motivation, realistic future plans. Family adjustment, feelings of security, identifications good. Great extent of goal and value differentiation, some feelings of conflict, high degree of self-insight. Self-esteem high. *Rated improved.*

Male. Perinatal stress: 0. SES: low. Educational stimulation: average. Emotional support: low.

Fairly active, friendly infant. Mother responsible, energetic, easygoing, patient. Cattell IQ 83; Vineland SQ 100. *At age 10*: WISC full-scale IQ 88, verbal IQ 79, performance IQ 101; Bender-Gestalt score 3. Psychologist notes extremely passive, immature behavior, neurotic defensiveness, fear. Parental conflict. *During adolescence*: Followed by Social Services. SCAT and STEP scores 25th to 55th percentile. *Interview ratings at age 18*: Mixed attitude toward school, content to get by. Realistic future plans. Poor social life and family adjustment. Weak feelings of family security, very rejecting father. Very great conflict feelings, some self-insight. Self-esteem low. *Rated unimproved*.

Male. Perinatal stress: 2. SES: low. Educational stimulation: low. Emotional support: average.

Very active infant; keeps to self; head-banging. Serious, solemn two-year-old. Mother affectionate, patient, kind. Cattell IQ 83; Vineland SQ 100. *At age 10*: WISC full-scale IQ 98, verbal IQ 89, performance IQ 108; Bender-Gestalt score 1. Grades D's and F's. Severe anxiety. Obsessive-compulsive defenses, severe repression. *During adolescence*: Contact with police because of two burglary incidents. SCAT and STEP scores 30th to 76th percentile. *Interview ratings at age 18*: Favorable attitude toward school, high achievement motivation, realistic future plans. Family adjustment very good, feelings of security and identifications strong. Some goal and value differentiation, some self-insight. Few conflict feelings. Self-esteem fair. *Rated improved*.

Male. Perinatal stress: 1. SES: very low. Educational stimulation and emotional support in home: very low.

Quiet infant, keeps to self, head-banging; dependent, restless, distractible, active two-year-old. Mother careless, childlike, easygoing, erratic. Cattell IQ 100; Vineland SQ 113. *At age 10*: WISC verbal IQ 125, performance IQ 87, full-scale IQ 108; Bender-Gestalt score 1. Perceptual-motor difficulties noted. Temper tantrums; "troublemaker"; persistent stealing and lying; destructive. D's and F's in reading, writing, arithmetic. *During adolescence*: SCAT and STEP scores 13th to 60th percentile. *Interview ratings at age 18*: Very unfavorable attitude toward school, low achievement motivation. Realistic future plans. Family adjustment poor, in conflict with parents. Little goal and value differentiation, little self-insight. Self-esteem very low. *Rated unimproved*.

Male. Perinatal stress: 1. SES: middle class. Educational stimulation and emotional support in home: low.

Affectionate infant, throws self down; disagreeable, insecure, restless, stubborn two-year-old. Mother complaining, fussy, childlike with infant; hostile, discontented with two-year-old. Cattell IQ 86; Vineland SQ 105. *At age 10*: WISC full-scale IQ 89, verbal IQ 84, performance IQ 97; Bender-Gestalt score 2. Repeated a grade. D's and F's in reading, writing, arithmetic. Anxious and depressed, nervous tremors. *During adolescence*: Followed by Public Health Nursing for orthopedic condition (corrective surgery done). Police report for minor larceny. SCAT and STEP scores 2nd to 19th percentile. *Interview ratings at age 18*: Very favorable attitude toward school, achievement motivation high. Future plans realistic. Family adjustment good, strong feelings of security and identifications. Goal and value differentiation great, little conflict, some self-insight. Self-esteem high. *Rated improved.*

Female. Perinatal stress: 0. SES: low. Educational stimulation and emotional support in home: low.

Very active, cuddly baby; holds breath. Stubborn, suspicious, solemn two-year-old. Mother matter-of-fact, reasonably relaxed, takes things in stride. Cattell IQ 100; Vineland SQ 120. *At age 10*: PMA IQ 98; Bender-Gestalt score 5. Frequent school absences, D's and F's in reading, writing, arithmetic. Stubborn, feelings easily hurt, tantrums. *During adolescence*: SCAT and STEP scores 1st to 28th percentile. School counselor-parent conferences regarding lack of interest. *Interview ratings at age 18*: Mixed attitude toward school, content to get by. Future plans realistic, social life and job satisfaction very good. Family adjustment, feelings of security, identifications very strong. Great degree of goal and value differentiation, little conflict, high degree of self-insight. Self-esteem very high. *Rated improved.*

Male. Perinatal stress: 0. SES: very low. Educational stimulation and emotional support in home: very low.

Fairly active infant, clings to mother; dependent, bashful, fearful, inhibited two-year-old. Mother indifferent, irresponsible, distant, hostile, childlike. Cattell IQ 74; Vineland SQ 91. *At age 10*: PMA IQ 95; Bender-Gestalt score 1. Grades D's and F's. Depressed, lacks self-confidence. Mother mentally ill. *During adoles-*

cence: Periodic contacts with Social Services. SCAT and STEP scores 26th to 76th percentile. *Interview ratings at age 18*: Unfavorable attitude toward school, content to get by. Somewhat unrealistic future plans. Very poor family adjustment, rejecting father, in conflict with mother. Goal and value differentiation very great. Some self-insight. Self-esteem fair. *Rated unimproved*.

Male. Perinatal stress: 1. SES: low. Educational stimulation: average. Emotional support: very low.

Fairly active infant; dislikes affection; head-banging. Tense, frustrated, serious two-year-old. Mother energetic, self-confident, intelligent, self-controlled with infant, but irritated with two-year-old. Cattell IQ 91; Vineland SQ 126. *At age 10*: WISC full-scale IQ 112, verbal IQ 104, performance IQ 118; Bender-Gestalt score 1. Grades D's and F's. Considered by psychologist as disorganized and aggressive; low frustration tolerance. Severe family problems including suicide attempts, alcoholism, divorce, parent death. Foster home placement. *During adolescence*: Known to school counselor, police, Family Court, Social Services. SCAT and STEP scores 6th to 27th percentile. *Interview ratings at age 18*: Favorable attitude toward school, content to get by. Adjustment in foster family fair. Adequate foster mother-son relationship; in conflict with foster father. Little goal and value differentiation, some conflict feelings, little self-insight. Self-esteem fair. *Rated unimproved*.

Female. Perinatal stress: 2. SES: low. Educational stimulation and emotional support in home: high.

Very active, affectionate infant; throws self on floor. Determined, eager, active, responsive, restless two-year-old. Mother stable, responsive, affectionate. Cattell IQ 105; Vineland SQ 142. *At age 10*: WISC full-scale IQ 88, verbal IQ 81, performance IQ 97; Bender-Gestalt score 0. Grades D's and F's. Daydreams, lacks confidence, emotionally immature. Extremely anxious, severe repression. *During adolescence*: Abortion at age 16. *Interview ratings at age 18*: Favorable attitude toward school, achievement motivation high. Future plans realistic. Family adjustment good, strong feelings of security and identifications. Great degree of goal and value differentiation, absence of conflict feelings, high degree of self-insight. Self-esteem high. *Rated improved*.

Male. Perinatal stress: 0. Educational stimulation: very low. Emotional support: low.

Fairly active, affectionate infant; head-banging. Insecure, withdrawn, uncommunicative two-year-old. Mother affectionate, takes things in stride, concerned. Cattell IQ 87; Vineland SQ 103. *At age 10*: Shy, distractible, temper tantrums, articulation difficulties. Diagnosis: schizoid personality development. Parental problems (drinking and fighting). *During adolescence*: Placed in Learning Center at school. Poor social adjustment. Vocational Rehabilitation referral requested by parent. (Left school at grade 11.) *Interview ratings at age 18*: Very unfavorable attitude toward school, dissatisfied with job. Poor family adjustment. Feels insecure. Rejected by father. Little goal and value differentiation. Very intense feelings of conflict. No self-insight. Self-esteem very low. *Rated unimproved.*

Female. Perinatal stress: 0. SES: low. Educational stimulation and emotional support in home: low.

Very active, cuddly infant; head-banging. Responsive, intelligent, independent, cheerful two-year-old. Mother affectionate, resourceful, mature, outgoing. Cattell IQ 116; Vineland SQ 153. *At age 10*: WISC full-scale IQ 103, verbal IQ 94, performance IQ 113; Bender-Gestalt score 6. Repeated year in school. Grades D's and F's. Psychologist notes fearful, constricted child. *During adolescence*: Parents divorced and remarried. *Interview ratings at age 18*: Content to get by in school, ambiguous future plans. Family adjustment and feelings of security fair. In conflict with parents. Some goal and value differentiation, some self-insight. Self-esteem fair. *Rated unimproved.*

Male. Perinatal stress: 0. SES: middle class. Educational stimulation and emotional support in home: average.

Fairly active, affectionate infant; dependent, restless, frustrated, uncommunicative two-year-old. Mother childlike, suggestible, indulgent. Cattell IQ 77; Vineland SQ 109. *At age 10*: PMA IQ 109; Bender-Gestalt score 7. Shy, daydreams, lacks self-confidence. *Interview ratings at age 18*: Mixed reactions toward school, adequate achievement motivation. Future plans realistic. Identifies strongly with parents, particularly father. Family adjustment good. Some goal and value differentiation, some conflict feelings. High degree of self-insight. Self-esteem fair. *Rated improved.*

Male. Perinatal stress: 1. SES: middle class. Educational stimulation and emotional support in home: low.

Very active infant; keeps to self. Active, agreeable, calm, independent two-year-old. Mother affectionate, stable, patient, mature. Cattell IQ 120; Vineland SQ 145. *At age 10*: WISC full-scale IQ 96, verbal IQ 91, performance IQ 103; Bender-Gestalt score 2. D's and F's in reading, writing, arithmetic. Psychologist notes constriction, repression, hostility, confusion. Death of father in childhood. *During early adolescence*: Contact with Mental Health at age 12. SCAT and STEP scores 1st to 17th percentile. *Interview ratings at age 18*: Favorable attitude toward school, content to get by. Relatively realistic future plans. Poor family adjustment, little goal and value differentiation. Some conflict feelings, no self-insight. Self-esteem very low. *Rated unimproved.*

Male. Perinatal stress: 0. SES: low. Educational stimulation and emotional support in home: low.

Very active infant; active, frustrated, responsive two-year-old. Mother kind, takes things in stride, reasonable, patient. Cattell IQ 96; Vineland SQ 117. *At age 10*: WISC full-scale IQ 95, verbal IQ 97, performance IQ 93; Bender-Gestalt score 4. Grades D's and F's. Very shy, concentration difficulties, immature. Nervous, anxious child. Unsupervised at home, neglected. *During adolescence*: School report of cutting classes, gambling; on academic probation. SCAT and STEP scores 3rd to 28th percentile. Known to police for "minor" attack on girl. Refused interview. Parent reported youth not doing anything after graduation. *Rated unimproved.*

Female. Perinatal stress: 0. SES: very low. Educational stimulation and emotional support in home: low.

Very active, affectionate infant; agreeable, independent, sociable two-year-old. Mother resourceful, warmhearted, easygoing, mildly ambivalent. Cattell IQ 100; Vineland SQ 117. *At age 10*: WISC full-scale IQ 91, verbal IQ 82, performance IQ 103; Bender-Gestalt score 1. Depressed, fearful; mind wanders; no signs of affection from significant adults. School grades D's and F's in reading, writing, arithmetic. *During adolescence*: Frequent school absences, gambling, aggressive behavior. Known to police and Family Court. SCAT and STEP scores 5th to 25th percentile. *Interview ratings at age 18*: Favorable attitude toward school, content to get by, realistic future plans. Very poor family adjustment, in conflict with mother, very rejecting father, very weak feelings of security. Some goal and value differentiation, very great conflict feelings, some self-insight. Self-esteem fair. *Rated unimproved.*

Female. Perinatal stress: 0. SES: very low. Educational stimulation and emotional support in home: very low.

Fairly active, affectionate infant; head-banging. Mother unintelligent, erratic, childlike, dependent. *At age 10*: WISC verbal IQ 69, performance IQ 97, full-scale IQ 80; Bender-Gestalt score 1. Grades D's and F's; repeated one grade. Depressed, irritable, pronounced shyness, considerable unrelieved tension and aggression. Responds explosively to threats and conflicts. Intense family problems and parental inadequacies. *During adolescence*: Aloof, hostile, defiant, runaway, foster home placement. Active with Family Court, Social Services, Mental Health. Brief psychiatric hospitalization, drug therapy, psychotherapy, diagnosis of borderline psychosis. Below-average schoolwork, dropped out before graduation. *Interview ratings at age 18 (questionnaire)*: Ambivalent about school, undecided regarding future plans. Family adjustment very poor, fairly strong parental identifications. *Rated unimproved.*

Four additional LMH children (two with a perinatal stress score of 0, one with a perinatal stress score of 1, and one with a perinatal stress score of 2) had incomplete follow-up data. One LMH child, with a perinatal stress score of 2, is among the LD's.

SMH Children

In this section we present brief synopses of children's behavior at age 10 which led to recommendation for short-term mental health services. Behavior was reported independently by parent, teacher, and/or psychologist.

Female. *Stepmother*: Temper tantrums; lacks self-confidence; extremely shy; feelings hurt easily; afraid of dark; frequent lying to keep out of trouble. *Teacher*: Extremely shy when it comes to classroom participation; seems to have difficulty adjusting to new home situation (father remarried, adding several children to family).

Male. *Father*: Very unhappy, depressed most of the time, especially after mother left family. Feelings hurt easily. *Teacher*: Lacks self-confidence; shy; has defeated attitude before he tries anything; does not participate in physical education, especially with other boys. Prefers to be with girls. Nervous habits; keeps shaking legs when seated; poor hand coordination.

Female. *Mother*: Inability to sit still; unable to concentrate, distractible. *Psychologist*: Poor self-concept, quite dissatisfied with self. Reports that mother "scolds a lot" and father "not around much." Needs supportive adult to talk to.

Male. *Mother*: Gets restless; bad temper; feelings hurt easily. *Teacher*: Lacks self-confidence; very shy; contributes very little to classroom discussion and that with reserve. *Psychologist*: Quiet, anxious, very tense; personality pattern of compulsive, anxious individual who is immature in capacity for emotional relationships and quite dependent on adult figures. Superego pressures quite strong, limit his inclination for assertive, exploratory behavior.

Male. *Mother*: Real problems with bed-wetting (two, three times a week) at age 10; very quiet, shy; feelings hurt easily, especially when older brother teases him; unable to concentrate; distractible. *Teacher*: Poor articulation in class; lack of self-confidence; unsure of self.

Female. *Mother*: Stuttered since age 3; unable to sit still since she is so nervous; temper tantrums since age 6; stamps feet, cries, throws things; lacks self-confidence; extremely shy; feelings hurt easily; quarrels with sister; when mad, destroys things on purpose. *Teacher*: Lacks self-confidence; shy, fearful, anxious.

Male. *Teacher*: Could do better in class; cannot get information for self; listens only to what interests him. *Psychologist*: Anxious, tense, too eager to please.

Female. *Mother*: Sucks thumb (at age 10); has temper tantrums; constantly quarreling; overaggressive; contrary and stubborn when she cannot have her way. *Teacher*: Unable to sit still in class; marked inability to concentrate; bullies; known to take sides in quarrels that do not concern her. *Psychologist*: Strong feeling of inadequacy and lack of self-confidence contribute to her uncommunicative behavior.

Female. *Mother*: Temper tantrums, uncontrolled emotions; overly contrary and stubborn; usually fights with two sisters because they tease her; when she gets mad, she slaps them.

Male. *Mother*: Most of the time he is trouble. Fights in school and with brothers; constantly quarreling, overaggressive; unable to sit still; lies frequently. *Teacher*: Easily frustrated and upset; uncontrolled emotions, temper tantrums; extremely irritable.

Male. *Mother*: Temper; gets mad quickly; fights with all his brothers; extremely irritable; extremely shy. *Psychologist*: Shy; lacks self-confidence; feels insecure.

Female. *Grandmother* (who legally adopted child): Bites nails; temper tantrums. *Teacher*: Marked inability to concentrate, distractible; tendency to push people around; slaps others if they don't listen to her.

Male. *Mother*: Nail-biting; staring spells; unable to concentrate; distractible; "mind wanders"; frequent lying.

Male. *Mother*: Used to stutter and stammer; now bites nails very badly. Temper tantrums, especially since father left family; seems to be against mother, seems bullyish and overaggressive; overly contrary and stubborn, gives mother a rough time. Has seen mother and father fight many times; on these occasions he is very calm and watches. *Teacher*: Extremely irritable; breaks rules of conduct; wants own way.

Female. *Mother*: Overaggressive; stubborn; destroys things on purpose; quick to punch and slap. *Teacher*: Attitude very poor; picks fights easily.

Male. *Mother*: Temper tantrums, uncontrolled emotions. *Teacher*: Unsure of self; anxious; lacks self-confidence; hesitant in speech.

Male. *Mother*: Nail-biting since age 8; temper tantrums since age 9; throws things when mad; feelings hurt easily.

Female. *Mother*: Sucks thumb; temper tantrums, uncontrolled emotions; afraid she might do something terrible in one of her outbursts; lacks self-confidence; feelings hurt easily; stubborn; "child is different."

Male. *Mother*: Drank from baby bottle till first grade; won't sleep alone at age 10; sleeps with sister; won't go from living room to bath alone; always moving around; unable to sit still; lacks self-confidence; gives up easily; depends on help in hard problems. *Psychologist*: Limited ego strength leads to overreaction in conflict situations; mild neurotic conflicts.

Female. *Mother*: Overly contrary and stubborn. *Psychologist*: Shy, rather schizoid personality; difficulties in interpersonal relationships and tends to feel threatened; handles feelings by repression and denial; somewhat tenuous hold on reality.

Female. *Mother*: Bites nails; feelings hurt easily; feels insecure. *Teacher*: Uncontrolled emotions; very immature; cries easily; thinks too much of her feelings.

Female. *Mother*: Bites nails; wets bed.

Male. *Mother*: Unable to sit still; fears dark; feelings hurt easily. *Teacher*: Hyperactive, unable to sit still; squirms; marked inability to concentrate; distractible. *Psychologist*: Anxious, confused, hostile; constricted by repressing hostile feelings.

Male. *Mother*: Lacks self-confidence; extremely shy; feelings hurt easily; depressed during father's absence; afraid father will leave him. *Teacher*: Seems in a dreamworld at times; mind wanders; has difficulty working by self for a period of time.

Male. *Mother*: Excitable, jumps around a lot and throws things; fidgets a lot; unable to concentrate, distractible; lacks self-confidence; extremely shy, feelings hurt easily; every once in a while locks self in and starts crying.

Female. *Mother*: Temper tantrums, uncontrolled emotions; screams and cries, fights with sisters; unable to concentrate, distractible; feelings hurt easily. *Teacher*: Marked inability to concentrate; quickly bored. *Psychologist*: Rather anxious and frightened girl who does not have an outlet for hostility other than passive resistance and foot-dragging; has much immature fantasy and escapes in a dreamworld whenever things become difficult or boring for her. Interpersonal relations seem unusually threatening to her.

Male. *Mother*: Stutters and stammers; bites nails; temper tantrums; feelings hurt easily; contrary and stubborn when he cannot get his way.

Male. *Grandmother* (adoptive parent): Quite a temper; hits playmates and brothers; throws things; feelings hurt easily; doesn't want to lose; destroys things on purpose when angry.

Male. *Mother*: Bites nails; extremely irritable; takes anger out on small children; very unhappy, depressed most of the time; lacks self-confidence. *Teacher*: Needs to develop self-confidence, self-control, direction.

Male. *Mother*: Bites nails; unable to sit still; unable to concentrate; mind seems to wander; very unhappy, depressed over school; feelings hurt easily; doesn't want to sleep in own bed; insists on sleeping with mother or father. *Teacher*: Marked inability to concentrate, distractible. *Psychologist*: Blunt and inhibited personality; much perseveration; flat affect.

Male. *Mother*: Unable to sit still; attention wanders; unable to concentrate; is a worrier, mostly about doing poorly in school; lacks self-confidence; feelings easily hurt. *Teacher*: Stutters and stammers; many nervous habits; uncontrolled temper. Unable to concentrate; lacks self-confidence; bullying; constantly quarreling; negativistic.

Male. *Mother*: Bites nails; finicky about eating; unable to sit still; uncontrolled emotions; hits and throws anything (including hammer at sister); distractible; extremely irritable; lacks self-confidence; feelings hurt easily; lies frequently, destroys things on purpose.

Male. *Mother*: Stutters, especially when excited; lisps; temper tantrums, uncontrolled emotions, extremely irritable; stubborn. *Teacher*: Some difficulty with stuttering.

Female. *Mother*: Bites nails; unable to concentrate; distractible; extremely irritable; gets angry very fast with playmates; extremely shy; feelings hurt very easily; overly contrary, stubborn. *Teacher*: Lisps; hunches up shoulders; very shy in class; bullying; quarreling out of class; lies frequently. *Psychologist*: Few adaptive defenses on the projective tests; seems to reject feminine identification and expresses anger in response to oral deprivation; appears tense, constricted.

Male. *Mother*: "As a baby he was very different from the other children." Gets mad quickly (from babyhood till present); feelings hurt easily ever since little; lies frequently.

Male. *Mother*: Wiggles nose; finicky about eating; unable to sit still; feelings hurt easily. *Teacher*: Stammers; squints, twitches facial muscles; unable to concentrate. *Psychologist*: Restrained, constrictive thinking reflects emotional problems; fantasies made up of yearning for simple affection and fear of retaliation for indiscretions.

Male. *Mother*: Unable to sit still; lies to keep out of trouble. *Teacher*: Twitches facial muscles; hyperactive; unable to sit still in class; easily distracted; truant from school.

Female. *Mother*: Nervous mannerisms (taps feet, clears throat); temper tantrums; screams and chokes brother; always fights with sister; constantly quarrels with siblings; afraid of dark.

Male. *Mother*: Sucked thumb till age 8, now bites nails; temper tantrums, uncontrolled emotions; afraid of rocking chairs, going downhill in a car; anxious, depressed; quarrels; contrary, stubborn; lies frequently; runs away from home.

Male. *Mother*: Unable to sit still; temper tantrums, uncontrolled emotions; when sisters or playmates tease him, he hits; always has to win; feelings hurt easily; lies frequently concerning schoolwork.

Male. *Mother*: Makes funny faces; wets lips so much they are sore; temper tantrums, uncontrolled emotions; screams and hits siblings when mad; feelings hurt easily; lies a lot; when mother tries to correct him, he says: "Nobody likes me; everybody picks on me." Mother thinks child needs help.

Female. *Mother*: Temper tantrums, uncontrolled emotions; screams, cries, throws things; extremely irritable; extremely shy; constantly quarreling. Contrary and stubborn; frequently lies about other people; does not make friends in school.

Female. *Mother*: Bites nails, wets bed; temper tantrums; would hold breath until she got blue to get what she wanted; when really angry will throw things at people. Very unhappy, depressed most of the time. *Teacher*: Family situation must be bothering her. *Psychologist*: Rather sensitive and dreamy youngster; expresses basic dissatisfaction with family situation (she lives presently with grandmother; mother, stepfather, sibs live nearby).

Female. *Mother*: Very sensitive child; lacks self-confidence, extremely shy; feelings easily hurt; cries easily when reprimanded; used to suck thumb. *Teacher*: Bites nails; when afraid or anxious can develop stomachache, nausea; keeps feelings to self; very shy and sensitive.

Female. *Mother*: Lacks self-confidence; is the worrying type. *Teacher*: Lacks self-confidence, pronounced shyness.

Female. *Mother*: Stutters, stammers; unable to sit still; throws things, bites; extremely irritable; feelings hurt easily; quarrels with older brother; slams door when angry, destroys things on purpose; mother has seen father make advances toward own daughter; daughter sleeps with mother. *Teacher*: Easily distracted; anxious about family's problems; overaggressive with younger children.

Female. *Teacher*: Lacks self-confidence; pronounced shyness. *Psychologist*: Tends to be shy and passive when more aggressive behavior would be appropriate; responds with considerable concern over failure and avoids potentially failure-producing situations.

Male. *Mother*: Tics, nervous clearing of throat, blinking; wets bed; unable to sit still; temper tantrums, uncontrolled emotions; gets quite angry at parents and sibs; bangs door and yells. *Teacher*: Afraid of being reprimanded; tends to withdraw.

Male. *Mother*: Bites nails; wets bed; finicky about eating; unable to sit still; uncontrolled emotions; throws and breaks things; afraid to go out at night. *Teacher*: Marked inability to concentrate, distractible; steals in class.

Female. *Mother*: Cannot sit still; uncontrolled emotions; screams and kicks; feelings hurt easily; cries easily. *Teacher*: Listless; extremely irritable with actions of other girls; lacks self-confidence; seems embarrassed; seems to delight in blaming others or getting them into trouble; truant from school.

Male. *Mother*: Lacks self-confidence, extremely shy; feelings hurt easily. *Psychologist*: Projective material suggests neurotic adjustment. Concerned with feelings which threaten to disorganize him; considerable energy spent controlling them. Evidence of considerable anxiety. Feels angry, depressed; preoccupied with powerful adult male figures.

Male. *Mother*: Bites nails. *Teacher*: Hyperactive, unable to sit still in class; negativistic; when corrected for error, throws away paper, sits and sulks; seems to seek recognition by bullying, aggressiveness, constant quarreling, especially on playground. *Psychologist*: Tense, constricted child.

Female. *Mother*: Terrible tantrums; gets mad easily, throws sister and things about; extremely irritable; cries easily; feelings hurt easily; contrary and stubborn; destroys things on purpose. *Psychologist*: Extremely self-conscious; easily frustrated; quite aware of intellectual limitations and tendency to be stubborn and irritable. Very dependent, afraid to grow up. Strong needs for nurturance only temporarily satisfied by material things; but always wants more because she seems to experience a deep sense of rejection. Quality of suspiciousness that might become serious.

Female. *Mother*: Bites nails; giggles to cover embarrassment; bashful child; feelings easily hurt; lacks self-confidence. *Teacher*: Sensitive child, cries easily in classroom.

Female. *Mother*: Sucked thumbs till age 7; temper tantrums; screams and hollers, throws things, even at mother; feelings hurt easily ever since little; can be contrary and stubborn; gets crying spells and headaches.

Female. *Mother*: Bites nails; temper tantrums, uncontrolled emotions; used to cry and cry to get what she wanted; now she throws things like brushes, knife; cries until lips get blue; destroys things on purpose when fighting with sister; overly contrary and stubborn.

Four SMH children (three with perinatal stress scores of 0 and one with a perinatal stress score of 1) are among the LD's.

APPENDIX 4
Instruments Used in the Follow-up

Novicki Locus of Control Scale

Name   _____

Date   _____

School   _____

Grade   _____

Directions: In each of the 40 items below check either YES or NO.

	YES*	NO*
1. Do you believe that most problems will solve themselves if you just don't fool with them?	X	_____
2. Do you believe that you can stop yourself from catching a cold?	_____	X
3. Are some people just born lucky?	X	_____
4. Most of the time do you feel that getting good grades meant a great deal to you?	_____	X
5. Are you often blamed for things that just aren't your fault?	X	_____
6. Do you believe that if somebody studies hard enough he or she can pass any subject?	_____	X

	YES*	NO*
7. Do you feel that most of the time it doesn't pay to try hard because things never turn out right anyway?	X	
8. Do you feel that if things start out well in the morning it's going to be a good day no matter what you do?	X	
9. Do you feel that most of the time parents listen to what their children have to say?		X
10. Do you believe that wishing can make good things happen?	X	
11. When you get punished does it usually seem it's for no good reason at all?	X	
12. Most of the time do you find it hard to change a friend's (mind) opinion?	X	
13. Do you think that cheering more than luck helps a team to win?		X
14. Did you feel that it was nearly impossible to change your parent's mind about anything?	X	
15. Do you believe that parents should allow children to make most of their own decisions?		X
16. Do you feel that when you do something wrong there's very little you can do to make it right?	X	
17. Do you believe that most people are just born good at sports?	X	
18. Are most of the other people your age stronger than you are?	X	
19. Do you feel that one of the best ways to handle most problems is just not to think about them?	X	
20. Do you feel that you have a lot of choice in deciding who your friends are?		X
21. If you find a four leaf clover, do you believe it might bring you good luck?	X	
22. Did you often feel that whether or not you did your homework had much to do with what kind of grades you got?		X
23. Do you feel that when a person your age is angry at you, there's little you can do to stop him or her?	X	
24. Have you ever had a good luck charm?	X	

	YES*	NO*
25. Do you believe that whether or not people like you depends on how you act?		X
26. Did your parents usually help you if you asked them to?		X
27. Have you felt that when people were angry with you it was usually for no reason at all?	X	
28. Most of the time, do you feel that you can change what might happen tomorrow by what you do today?		X
29. Do you believe that when bad things are going to happen they just are going to happen no matter what you try to do to stop them?	X	
30. Do you think people can get their own way if they just keep trying?		X
31. Most of the time do you find it useless to try to get your own way at home?	X	
32. Do you feel that when good things happen they happen because of hard work?		X
33. Do you feel that when somebody your age wants to be your enemy there's little you can do to change matters?	X	
34. Do you feel that it's easy to get friends to do what you want them to do?		X
35. Do you usually feel that you have little to say about what you get to eat at home?	X	
36. Do you feel that when someone doesn't like you there's little you can do about it?	X	
37. Did you usually feel that it was almost useless to try in school because most other children were just plain smarter than you are?	X	
38. Are you the kind of person who believes that planning ahead makes things turn out better?		X
39. Most of the time, do you feel that you have little to say about what your family decides to do?	X	
40. Do you think it's better to be smart than to be lucky?		X

*Checkmarks denote scoring key for Novicki Locus of Control Scale.

Interview, Questionnaire, and Interview Ratings

INTERVIEW

Name   _____
School   _____
Code No.   _____
Interviewer   _____
Date   _____

A. INTERESTS AND ACTIVITIES

1. *Lead Question*: I want to talk first with you about the things you're interested in and what kinds of activities you like to do.

2. What activities do you like to do most of all (including extra-curricular at school)?

3. Do you belong to any clubs or other organizations?

B. SCHOOL

4. *Lead Question*: Would you give me some of your impressions and feelings about high school?

5. How satisfied were you with the education you received during high school? Reasons?

6. Were you pretty satisfied with the way you did in school?

7. How important was it to you to do well in school? Why?

C. EDUCATION AND OCCUPATIONAL PLANS

8. *Lead Question*: I am interested in what you would like to be doing in the future and whether you think you will be able to do it.

9. How far do you plan to go in school or college? Why have you decided that (reasons for whatever decision)?

10. Have you decided what kind of work you want to do when you finish school (college)? Why do you think you want to go into it?

11. For girls only: Do you plan to work or to get married, or both?

12. If planning both career and marriage: Do you think you will want to work after you have children? Which do you think will be more important to you— your work or your marriage and family?

D. WORK

13. *Lead Question*: Do you work now? Could you tell me something about the kind of work you are doing? Full time: Part time:

14. Why are you working? What do you feel are some important characteristics about your future job?

E. RELATIONS WITH FRIENDS

15. *Lead Question*: With whom do you spend most of your time?

16. Now tell me something about your friends. Do you most enjoy doing things with a group, with one or two friends, or by yourself?

17. How well do you get along with other people? How well do they like you?

18. What kind of people do you not like to associate with?

19. What kind of people do you look up to?

20. Do you have a girlfriend or a friend? Do you feel like telling me anything about it?

F. FAMILY

21. *Lead Question*: Now tell me something about your family. Do you have any brothers or sisters (ages and relationship)? Do you live with your parents now? If not, then how long have you been away and why? With whom do you live now?

22. What kinds of things do you do together as a family?

23. What is your mother like?

24. What is your father like?

25. How do you get along with your parents presently?

26. How close do you feel to your mother? Do you feel you are like your mother in any way?

27. How close do you feel to your father? Do you feel you are like your father in any way?

28. How well do you feel your parents understand you?

29. Parents influence their children in different ways. How do you think your mother has influenced you? How much do you and your mother talk?

30. Your father—has he influenced you? How much do you and your father talk?

31. Who is the main parent in your family who has had the most to do with you being the way you are now?

32. What did your parents stress when you were growing up?

33. What did they want you to be? Mother: _____. Father:_____. How far will they support you (if in college)?

34. How do you think your parents got ideas of right and wrong and how to be a good person across to you? How did they go about it?

35. What kind of rules do you have in your family? Who makes them? How are they enforced?

36. All families have disagreements but they differ in how they show it and what they do about it. What's it like in your family?

37. How much does your family talk to you about things that concern you? Which parent are you likely to talk things over with?

38. What other members of your family had a major influence on you? Who? Why? What about your brothers and sisters?

G. SELF

39. Now let's talk a little bit about you. How has your health been? Do you take any medication?

40. What do you feel are your strong points and weak points? Are there any ways in which you are trying to change or develop yourself?

41. Do you have any special goals or objectives (either short term or long range) that you are working toward?

42. What do you most want to achieve in life? (When you think ahead, what do you most want to get out of life?) If "happiness" or similar answer: How do you think you are most likely to achieve this?

43. Everybody worries about some things; what kinds of things worry you? What about new experiences—getting into situations you haven't been in before—do you worry about these?

44. Have you ever gotten help from another when you had a problem? Who? If no: Have you ever thought about it?

45. What was the problem for which you sought help?

46. What do you feel you gained from this experience?

47. Over what period of time and how often did you see the counselor?

48. Was it alone or with your family?

49. Why did you stop?

50. If you never got help, was there a time you considered it or thought you might need it?

51. What are the most important experiences and influences that have helped make you the kind of person you are? (Have particular people or experiences been important in shaping your outlook and personality?)

52. Is there anything you feel is important to you that we haven't talked about?

Additional questions on drugs, sex, race.

QUESTIONNAIRE

Name   _____
Code No.   _____
(Fill in before mailing)

1.   What activities do you like to do most of all? Check:

____   1. Sports. Specify: _____
____   2. Watching TV.
____   3. Movies.
____   4. Playing musical instruments. Specify: _____
____   5. Arts in general.
____   6. Crafts.
____   7. Church group activities.
____   8. Listening to music.
____   9. Rapping with friends.
____   10. Reading.
____   11. Hiking, camping, outdoor life.
____   12. Political work.
____   13. Parties.
____   14. School-related organizations. _____
____   15. Non-school-related organizations. _____
____   16. Family recreation. Specify: _____
____   17. Other. Specify: _____

2.   How far do you plan to go in school or college?

____   1. Less than high school graduation.
____   2. High school graduation.
____   3. Technical training beyond high school (airplane mechanic, drama, secretarial, etc.).
____   4. Junior college. Specify:_____
____   5. Four-year college. Specify: _____
____   6. Graduate school. Specify: _____
____   7. Other. Specify: _____
____   8. Undecided.

3.   Have you decided what kind of work you want to do when you finish school?

____   1. Undecided.
____   2. Police.
____   3. Law, medicine, dentistry.
____   4. Tourist related. Specify: _____
____   5. Teaching.
____   6. Small business. Specify: _____
____   7. Farming, ranching, plantation work.
____   8. Military.

____   9. National or international service: Peace Corps, Vista.
____ 10. Nursing, dental hygiene.
____ 11. Clerical, office work, secretarial, cashier.
____ 12. Skilled trade: carpentry, electrician, sheet metal, auto mechanic.
____ 13. Business and retail selling—department store.

4.   Why do you think you want to go into that kind of work?

____   1. Hours worked (schedule).
____   2. Change to express self.
____   3. Little tension, stress.
____   4. Good income.
____   5. Interesting work.
____   6. Benefit to society.
____   7. Opportunity for advancement.
____   8. Freedom from supervision.
____   9. Chance to meet and be with people.
____ 10. Use of skill and abilities.
____ 11. Respect others give to job.
____ 12. Freedom to develop own ideas.
____ 13. Security.

5.   How satisfied are you with the high school education you were getting?

____   1. Very much dissatisfied.
____   2. More dissatisfied than satisfied.
____   3. Ambivalent, somewhat satisfied and somewhat dissatisfied.
____   4. On the whole satisfied.
____   5. Very well satisfied.

6.   How important is it for you to do well in school?

____   1. No importance, don't care.
____   2. Little importance.
____   3. Some importance.
____   4. High importance.

7.   What kind of work are you doing now?

____   1. Have never worked for pay.
____   2. Babysitting; paper route.
____   3. Yard work; housework.
____   4. Summer camp.
____   5. Help in family business.
____   6. Commercial and industrial (waitress, gas station, cannery, etc.).
____   7. Plantation work.

8.   Why are you working?

____   1. Have never worked.

____ 2. Want money.
____ 3. Want experience.
____ 4. Interest.

9. With whom do you spend most of your time?

____ 1. No closest friend.
____ 2. One closest friend.
____ 3. Two or more very close friends.
____ 4. Parent.
____ 5. Other family member.

10. What about dating?

____ 1. Have had steady boyfriend or girlfriend, but do not currently have one.
____ 2. Steady boyfriend or girlfriend—still see other members of opposite sex.
____ 3. Very steady, exclusive arrangement.
____ 4. Engaged or plan to be married.
____ 5. Married.
____ 6. Marriage terminated.

11. Do you live with your parents now? Yes: ____. No: ____. If not, with whom do you live?

____ 1. Living with both natural parents.
____ 2. Living with natural mother only.
____ 3. Living with natural father only.
____ 4. Living with natural mother and stepfather.
____ 5. Living with natural father and stepmother.
____ 6. Others. Specify: _____

12. How would you describe your parents, using this series of adjectives? Check:

	Mother	Father			Mother	Father
Optimistic				Pessimistic		
Reserved				Outgoing		
Relaxed				Tense		
Often angry				Seldom angry		
Accepting				Critical		
Undemonstrative				Affectionate		
Dominant				Submissive		
Shy				Not shy		
High energy				Low energy		
Timid				Daring		
Competitive				Not competitive		
Unhappy				Happy		

13.   Parents tend to have goals for their children or qualities that they consider as especially important. Mark below the *three* qualities most important to your mother and the *three* qualities most important to your father:

	Mother (Most Important)	Father (Most Important)
That I be popular		
That I have good manners		
That I be ambitious		
That I be liked by adults		
That I act in a serious way		
That I be able to defend myself		
That I have self-control		
That I be affectionate		
That I be independent		
That I obey my parents well		
That I be honest		
That I be dependable		
That I be considerate of others		
That I be curious about things		
That I be a good student		
That I be neat and clean		
That I be successful in my job		

14.   When you were growing up (check the column that applies):

	Father Much More	Father Somewhat More	Both About Same	Mother Somewhat More	Mother Much More
1. Which parent was easiest to talk to?					
2. Which parent do you resemble most in personality?					
3. Which parent is the model for the kind of person you would like to be?					
4. Which parent were you most likely to discuss problems with?					

	Father Much More	Father Somewhat More	Both About Same	Mother Somewhat More	Mother Much More
5. Which parent understands you best as an individual?					
6. Which parent was more eager for you to do good work at school?					
7. Which parent was more likely to support you in the things you wanted to do?					
8. Which parent showed you the most affection?					

15. What does your family do when you disagree on something?

_____ 1. Family never has disagreements to speak of.
_____ 2. Family argues and discusses with no resolution; family go their separate ways.
_____ 3. Children's disagreeing viewpoint is listened to, but then the parents make the decision and tell the children.
_____ 4. Family discusses the disagreement and usually arrives at a decision that is reasonably acceptable to all parties.
_____ 5. Family fights and/or argues with no resolution.

16. How much does your family as a whole talk together about things that concern members?

_____ 1. Little discussion within family.
_____ 2. Some discussion, but rather haphazard.
_____ 3. Considerable tendency to talk together.

17. What kind of rules and regulations do you have in your family?

_____ 1. No rules.
_____ 2. Household chores.
_____ 3. My personal appearance.
_____ 4. Hour of coming in.
_____ 5. Letting parents know where I am.
_____ 6. Use of car.
_____ 7. Homework.
_____ 8. Watching TV.
_____ 9. Grades to be achieved.
_____ 10. My friends.
_____ 11. Other. Specify: _____

18. Who makes the rules in your home?

____ 1. Parents set rules without consulting children.
____ 2. Rules made by parents, but children at least consulted.
____ 3. Rules mutually arrived at by children and parents.
____ 4. Other. Specify: _____

19. What do you consider your strong points? More than one may be checked.

____ 1. Aggressiveness—gets in there and tries.
____ 2. Good nature, even temper.
____ 3. Understanding—good listener.
____ 4. Honesty.
____ 5. Hardworking—perserverance.
____ 6. Patience.
____ 7. Loyalty.
____ 8. Intellectual interests.
____ 9. Looks.
____ 10. Athletic ability.
____ 11. Special talent (art, music, etc.) Specify:_____
____ 12. Academic achievement.
____ 13. Other. Specify: _____

20. What do you consider your weak points? More than one may be checked.

____ 1. Selfishness.
____ 2. Laziness.
____ 3. Not a good student.
____ 4. Bad-tempered.
____ 5. Domineering—willful.
____ 6. Weak—doesn't stand up for self.
____ 7. Lacks self-confidence.
____ 8. Undecided—confused.
____ 9. Looks, body build.
____ 10. Negative attitude.
____ 11. Other. Specify: _____

21. What do you most want to achieve in life?

____ 1. Helpfulness to others, social concern.
____ 2. Close, open relationships with friends, many friends, etc.
____ 3. Self-fulfillment, self-expression.
____ 4. Self-improvement, working to increase skills, relationships, become less difficult, less despondent, etc.
____ 5. Be a moral person, "good Christian," other statements suggesting high moral caliber as ideal.
____ 6. Happiness as end in self (have a good time, enjoy life, etc.).
____ 7. Happy, successful marriage.
____ 8. Other. List:_____
____ 9. Career or job success.

22. Everyone worries about something; what kind of things worry you?

_____ 1. No worries.
_____ 2. Grades or school.
_____ 3. My future. Specify: _____
_____ 4. Parent's marriage.
_____ 5. State of the world.
_____ 6. Friends.
_____ 7. Money.
_____ 8. Sibling(s).
_____ 9. Opinions of others.
_____ 10. Other. Specify: _____

23. Have you gotten help from another when you had a problem? Yes: _____. No: _____. Who?

_____ 1. Older friends.
_____ 2. Peer friends.
_____ 3. Parent.
_____ 4. Teacher.
_____ 5. Counselor.
_____ 6. Other professionals. Specify: _____
_____ 7. Minister.

24. What was the problem for which you sought help?

25. When you think of the various influences on you at the present time—people whose ideas and opinions mean most to you—how would you rate each of the following? (Leave blank any that do not apply.)

				Influence on You	
	None(1)	Some(2)	Little Strong(3)	Very Strong(4)	Strongest(5)
Your father					
Your mother					
Brothers and sisters					
Closest friend—same sex					
Closest friend—opposite sex					
Friends in general					
Clergyman, priest, rabbi					
Teachers					
Other special persons. Who?					

26. To sum up: How would you describe yourself as a person?

ADOLESCENT INTERVIEW RATINGS

Overall attitude toward school
very favorable favorable mixed reactions unfavorable very unfavorable

Achievement motivation
very high   high   content to get by   low   very low

Participation in school activities (including extracurricular)
very extensive   extensive   some   limited   very limited

Realism of educational plans beyond high school
very realistic   realistic   mixed elements   unrealistic   very unrealistic

Job satisfaction (if applicable)
very satisfied   satisfied   ambivalent   dissatisfied   very dissatisfied

Social life (overall social adjustment)
very good   good   fair   poor   very poor

Feeling of security as part of family
very strong   strong   fair   weak   very weak

Identification with mother
identifies strongly   identifies   in conflict   rejecting   very rejecting

Identification with father
identifies strongly   identifies   in conflict   rejecting   very rejecting

Overall family adjustment
very good   good   fair   poor   very poor

Degree of self-insight
very high   high   some insight   little   none

Extent of goal differentiation
very great   great   some   little   none

Intensity of conflict feelings
very great   great   some   little   none

Self-esteem
very high   high   fair   low   very low

Interviewer's impression of conditions of interview
optimal   good   average   detrimental   seriously detrimental

Table 49   Reliability Coefficients Derived from Scores Given by
Interviewer and Three Other Raters to 13 Taped Interviews

Dimension	Reliability for Mean Ratings from 4 Raters	Reliability for Interviewer against Mean of 3 Other Raters
Overall attitude to school	.92	.84
Achievement motivation	.94	.92
Participation in school activities	.93	.90
Realism of educational plans	.83	.88
Job satisfaction	.89	.81
Social life	.81	.74
Feeling of security as part of family	.97	.93
Identification with mother	.96	.84
Identification with father	.95	.94
Overall family adjustment	.96	.91
Degree of self-insight	.81	.67
Extent of goal differentiation	.89	.83
Intensity of conflict feelings	.83	.77
Self-esteem	.73	.49
Ability to establish relationship in interview	.82	.67

References

Alberman, Eva. 1973. The early prediction of learning disorders. *Developmental Medicine and Child Neurology* **15**:202–204.

Anderson, J. E.; Harris, D. B.; Werner, E.; and Gallistel, E. 1959. *A survey of children's adjustment over time*. Minneapolis: Institute of Child Development.

Arkoff, Abe, and Leton, Donald A. 1966. Ethnic and personality patterns in college entrance. *Journal of Experimental Education* **35**:79–85.

Benaron, H. B. W.; Tucker, B. E.; Andrews, J. P.; Boshes, B.; Cohen, J.; Fromm, E.; and Yacorzynski, G. K. 1960. Effects of anoxia during labor and immediately after birth on the subsequent development of the child. *American Journal of Obstetrics and Gynecology* **54**:1129–1142.

Benjamin, Jeanette Ann. 1969. A study of the social psychological factors related to the academic success of Negro high school students. Unpublished Ph.D. dissertation, Northwestern University.

Berendes, H. W. 1966. The structure and scope of the Collaborative Project on cerebral palsy, mental retardation and other neurological and sensory disorders of infancy and childhood. In S. S. Chipman, A. N. Lilienfeld, B. G. Greenberg, and J. F. Donley (eds.), *Research methodology and needs in perinatal studies*. Springfield, Ill.: Thomas.

Berrien, F. K.; Arkoff, A.; and Iwahara, S. 1967. Generational differences in values: Americans, Japanese-Americans and Japanese. *Journal of Social Psychology* **71**:169–175.

Block, J. 1971. *Lives through time*. Berkeley: Bancroft Books.

Boggs, J. 1968. Adolescent girls in Aina Pumehana. Unpublished paper, University of Hawaii.

Brislin, R. W.; Lonner, W. J.; and Thorndike, R. M. 1973. *Cross-cultural research methods*. New York: Wiley.

Broman, S. H.; Nichols, P. L.; and Kennedy, W. A. 1975. Preschool IQ: Prenatal and early development correlates. New York, Wiley.

Brunswick, A. F. 1971. Adolescent health, sex and fertility. *American Journal of Public Health* **61**:711–728.

Cattell, P. 1940. *The measurement of intelligence of infants*. New York: Psychological Corporation.

Caudill, W., and DeVos, G. 1961. Achievement, culture and personality: The case of the Japanese-Americans. In Yehudi A. Cohen (ed.), *Social structure and personality*. New York: Holt.

Chess, S., and Thomas, A. 1969. Differences in outcome with early intervention in children with behavior disorders. In M. Roff and D. Ricks (eds.), *Life history research in psychopathology*. Minneapolis: University of Minnesota Press.

Cole, J. K. and Magnussen, M. G. 1967. Family situation factors related to remainers and terminators of treatment. *Psychotherapy* **4**:107–109.

Coleman, J. S. 1966. *Equality of educational opportunity*. Washington: U.S. Office of Education.

Cowen E. 1973. Social and community interventions. *Annual Review of Psychology* **24**:423–460.

D'Angelo, R., and Walsh, J. F. 1967. An evaluation of various therapy approaches with lower socio-economic group children. *Journal of Psychology* **67**:59–64.

Denhoff, E. 1973. The natural life history of children with minimal brain dysfunction. *Annals: New York Academy of Sciences*, 188–205.

Deutsch, Cynthia. 1973. Social class and child development. In B. Caldwell and H. Ricciuti (eds.), *Review of child development research, child development and social policy*. Vol. 3. Chicago: University of Chicago Press.

DeVos, G. 1968. Achievement and innovation in culture and personality. In E. Norbeck, G. Price-Williams, and W. McCorde (eds.), *The study of personality: An interdisciplinary appraisal*. New York: Holt.

———. (ed.). 1973. *Socialization for achievement: Essays on the cultural psychology of Japanese*. Berkeley: University of California Press.

Dixon, Paul W.; Fukuda, Nobuko K.; and Berens, Anne E. 1968. The influence of ethnic grouping on SCAT, teachers' ratings, and rank in high school. *Journal of Social Psychology* **75**(2):285–286.

———. 1970. Cognitive and personalogical factor patterns for Japanese-American high school students in Hawaii. *Psychologia: An International Journal of Psychology in the Orient* **13**(1):35–41.

Doll, E. A. 1953. *Measurement of social competence*. Minneapolis: Educational Testing Bureau.

Douglas, J. W. B. 1964. *The home and the school*. London: MacGibbon & Kee.

Dykman, R.; Peters, J.; and Ackerman, P. 1973. Experimental approaches to the study of minimal brain dysfunction: A follow-up study. *Annals: New York Academy of Sciences*, 93–108.

Fenz, Walter D., and Arkoff, Abe. 1962. Comparative need patterns of five ancestry groups in Hawaii. *Journal of Social Psychology* 58:67–89.

French, F.; Connor, A.; Bierman, J. M.; Simonian, K.; and Smith, R. S. 1968. Congenital and acquired handicaps of 10 year olds: Report of a follow-up study, Kauai, Hawaii. *American Journal of Public Health* 58:1388–1395.

Fricker, S. Machida, and Werner, E. 1976. Achievement orientation of adolescent women of Hawaiian, Japanese and Filipino-American descent. *Catalog of Selected Documents in Psychology.*

Fuchs, Lawrence H. 1961. *Hawaii pono: A social history.* New York: Harcourt Brace Jovanovich.

Gallimore, R. 1969. Variations in the motivation antecedent of achievement among Hawaii's ethnic groups. Paper presented at the conference on Culture and Mental Health in Asia and the Pacific, Honolulu.

Gallimore, R.; Boggs, J. W.; and Jordan, C. E. 1974. *Culture, behavior, and education: A study of Hawaiian-Americans.* Beverly Hills: Sage Publications.

Gallimore, R. and Howard, A. (eds.). 1968. *Studies in a Hawaiian community: Na makamako o Nanakuli.* Honolulu: Bernice P. Bishop Museum, Pacific Anthropological Records, Department of Anthropology.

Glavin, J. P. 1972. Persistence of behavior disorders in children. *Exceptional Children,* January: 367–376.

Gluck, M. R.; Tanner, M. M.; Sullivan, D. F.; and Erickson, P. A. 1964. A follow-up evaluation of 55 child guidance cases. *Behavioral Research and Therapy* 2:131–134.

Gordon, C. P., and Gallimore, R. 1972. Teacher ratings of behavior problems of Hawaiian American adolescents. *Journal of Cross-Cultural Psychology* 3:209–213.

Gough, H. 1969. *California psychological inventory manual.* Rev. ed. Palo Alto: Consulting Psychologists Press.

Gough, H.; DeVos, G.; and Mizushima, K. 1968. Japanese validation of the CPI social maturity index. *Psychological Reports* 22:143–146.

Griffith, Thomas. 1974. On the delicate subject of inequality. *Time,* 15 April.

Guthrie, George M., and Jacobs, Pepita J. 1966. *Child rearing and personality development in the Philippines.* University Park: Pennsylvania State University Press.

Havighurst, R. J.; Bowman, P. H.; Liddle, G. P.; Mathews, C. V.; and Pierce, C. V. 1962. *Growing up in River City.* New York: Wiley.

Hinton, G. G. 1963. Childhood psychosis or mental retardation? *Journal of the Canadian Medical Association* 89:1020–1024.

Horinouchi, I. 1967. Education values and pre-adaption in the acculturation of Japanese-Americans. *Sacramento Anthropological Society Papers* 7.

Horowitz, F. D., and Paden, L. Y., 1973. The effectiveness of environmental intervention programs. In B. Caldwell and H. Ricciuti (eds.), *Review of child development research, child development and social policy.* Vol. 3. Chicago: University of Chicago Press.

Howard, A.; Heighton, R.; Jordan, C.; and Gallimore, R. 1970. Traditional and modern adoption patterns in Hawaii. In V. Carroll (ed.), *Adoption in Eastern Oceania.* Honolulu: University of Hawaii Press.

Johnson, K. G.; Donnelly, J. H.; Scheble, R.; Wine, R. J.; and Weitzman, M. 1971. Survey of adolescent drug use: Sex and grade distribution. *American Journal of Public Health* 61:2418-2432.

Jones, M. C.; Bayley, N.; Macfarlane, J.; and Honzik, M. P. (eds.). 1971. *The course of human development.* Waltham, Mass.: Xerox College Publishing.

Kagan, J. 1964. American longitudinal research. *Child Development* 35:1-32.

Kagan, J., and Moss, H. A. 1962. *Birth to maturity.* New York: Wiley.

Kane, F. J., and Lachenbruch, P. 1973. Adolescent pregnancy: A study of aborters and non-aborters. *American Journal of Orthopsychiatry* 43(5):796-803.

Keeve, J. P.; Schlesinger, E. R.; Wight, B. W.; and Adams, P. 1969. Fertility experience of juvenile girls: A community-wide ten year study. *American Journal of Public Health* 59:2185-2198.

King, S. H. 1972. Coping and growth in adolescence. *Seminars in Psychiatry* 4(4):355-366.

Kitano, H. 1961. Differential child-rearing attitudes between first and second generation Japanese in the United States. *Journal of Social Psychology* 53:13-19.

———. 1969. *Japanese Americans: The evolution of a subculture.* Englewood Cliffs, N.J.: Prentice-Hall.

Knobloch, H., and Pasamanick, B. 1962. Etiological factors in early infantile autism and childhood schizophrenia. Paper presented at the 10th International Congress of Pediatrics, Lisbon.

———. 1966. Prospective studies on the epidemiology of reproductive casualty: Methods, findings and some implications. *Merrill-Palmer Quarterly* 12:27-43.

Kohlberg, L.; LaCross, J.; and Ricks, D. 1972. The predictability of adult mental health from childhood behavior. In B. B. Wolman (ed.), *Manual of child psychopathology.* New York: McGraw-Hill.

Koppitz, Elisabeth. 1964. *The Bender-Gestalt test for young children.* New York: Grune & Stratton.

Kraus, Philip E. 1973 *Yesterday's children: A longitudinal study of children from kindergarten into the adult years.* New York: Wiley.

Kubany, Edward S.; Gallimore, Ronald; and Buell, Judith. 1970. The effects of extrinsic factors on achievement-oriented behavior: A non-Western case. *Journal of Cross-Cultural Psychology* 1(1):77-84.

Lane, E. A., and Albee, G. W. 1966. The comparative birthweights of adult schizophrenics and their siblings. *Journal of Psychology* 64:227-231.

Langner, T. S. 1974. Family research project: welfare (AFDC) sample. Year 1 data: Summary of findings and comparison with cross-section sample. Unpublished progress report, Columbia University, Faculty of Medicine.

Laufer, M. 1971. Long-term management and some follow-up findings on the use of drugs with minimal cerebral syndromes. *Journal of Learning Disabilities* 4:55-59.

Lefcourt, H. M. 1966. Internal versus external control of reinforcement: A review. *Psychological Bulletin* 65:206-220.

Levitt, E. 1971. Research on psychotherapy with children. In A. E. Bergen and S. L. Garfield (eds.), *Handbook of psychotherapy and behavior change*. New York: Wiley.

Lewis, W. W. 1965. Continuity and intervention in emotional disturbance: A review. *Exceptional Children* 31:465-475.

Lind, Andrew W. 1967. *Hawaii's people*. 3rd ed. Honolulu: University of Hawaii Press.

Lipman-Blumen, J. 1972. How ideology shapes women's lives. *Scientific American* 226(1):34-42.

Lynn, D. B. 1974. *The father: His role in child development*. Monterey: Brooks/Cole.

Maccoby, M., and Modiano, N. 1966. On culture and equivalence. In J. S. Bruner, R. R. Olver, and P. M. Greenfield (eds.), *Studies in cognitive growth*. New York: Wiley.

Macfarlane, J. W.; Allan, L.; and Honzik, M. P. 1954. *A developmental study of the behavior problems of normal children between 21 months and 14 years*. Berkeley and Los Angeles: University of California Press.

Maloney, Michael P. 1968. The question of achievement in the Japanese American: A comment on cross-cultural research. *Psychologia: An International Journal of Psychology in the Orient* 11(3-4):143-158.

Mason, E. P. 1967. Comparison of personality characteristics of junior high school students from American Indian, Mexican, and Caucasian ethnic backgrounds. *Journal of Social Psychology* 73:145-155.

Masterson, J. F., Jr. 1967. *The psychiatric dilemma of adolescence*. Boston: Little Brown.

McClelland, D. C. 1961. *The achieving society*. Princeton, N.J.: Van Nostrand.

McNassor, D., and Hongo, R. 1972. *Strangers in their own land: Self-disparagement in ethnic Hawaiian youth on the island of Hawaii*. Mimeographed. Claremont College, Department of Education.

Mednick, S., and Schulsinger, F. 1969. Factors related to breakdown in children at high risk for schizophrenia. In M. Roff and D. Ricks (eds.), *Life history research in psychopathology*. Minneapolis: University of Minnesota Press.

Meier, John. 1973. Screening and assessment of young children at developmental risk. President's Committee on Mental Retardation. Washington: Government Printing Office.

Mendelson, W.; Johnson, N.; and Stewart, M. A. 1971. Hyperactive children as teenagers: A follow-up study. *Journal of Nervous and Mental Disease* 153(1):273–279.

Menkes, M. M.; Rowe, J. S.; and Menkes, J. H. 1967. A twenty-five-year follow-up study of the hyperkinetic child with minimal brain dysfunction. *Pediatrics* 39:393–399.

Meredith, G. 1965. Observations on the acculturation of Sansei Japanese-Americans in Hawaii. *Psychologia: An International Journal of Psychology in the Orient* 8:41–49.

Meredith, G., and Meredith, C. G. W. 1966. Acculturation and personality among Japanese-American college students in Hawaii. *Journal of Social Psychology* 68(first half): 175–182.

Minde, K.; Weiss, G.; and Mendelson, N. 1972. A 5-year follow-up study of 91 hyperactive school children. *Journal of the American Academy of Child Psychiatry* 11(3):595–610.

Minskoff, G. 1973. Differential approaches to prevalence estimates of learning disabilities. *Annals: New York Academy of Sciences*, 139–145.

Mizushima, K., and DeVos, G. 1967. An application of the California Psychological Inventory in the study of Japanese delinquency. *Journal of Social Psychology* 71:45–51.

Novicki, S. 1971. Correlates of locus of control in secondary school population. *Developmental Psychology* 4:477–478.

Novicki, S., and Duke, M. P. 1972. A locus of control scale for adults: An alternative to the Rotter. *Journal of Consulting and Clinical Psychology*.

Novicki, S., and Segal, B. 1974. Perceived parental characteristics, locus of control orientation and behavioral correlates of locus of control. *Developmental Psychology* 10:33–37.

Nydegger, William, and Nydegger, Corrine. 1966. *Tarong: An Ilocos barrio in the Philippines*. New York: Wiley.

Offer, D. 1969. *The psychological world of the teenager*. New York: Basic Books.

Onondaga County School Studies. 1964. *Persistence of emotional disturbances reported among second and fourth grade children*. Interim Report No. 1. Syracuse, N.Y.: Mental Health Research Unit (L. McCaffrey, J. Cumming, and B. Pawley).

Oppel, W., and Royston, A. B. 1971. Teenage births: Some social, psychological and physical sequelae. *American Journal of Public Health* 61:751–756.

Paine, R. W.; Werry, J. S.; and Quay, H. C. 1968. A study of minimal cerebral dysfunction. *Developmental Medicine and Child Neurology* 10:505–520.

Pasamanick, B.; Rogers, M. E.; and Lilianfeld, A. M. 1956. Pregnancy experience and the development of behavior disorders in children. *American Journal of Psychiatry* 112:613–618.

Pasamanick, B., and Knobloch, H. 1960. Brain damage and reproduction casualty. *American Journal of Orthopsychiatry* 30:298–305.

Pollack, M.; Woerner, M.; and Klein, D. 1969. A comparison of childhood characteristics of schizophrenics, personality disorders, and their siblings. In M. Roff and D. Ricks (eds.), *Life history research in psychopathology*. Minneapolis: University of Minnesota Press.

Robins, L. 1966. *Deviant children grown up*. Baltimore: Williams & Wilkins.

――――. 1970. Follow-up studies of behaviour disorders in children. In E. H. Hare and J. K. Wing (eds.), *Psychiatric epidemiology*. Nuffield Provincial Hospital Trusts.

Roen, S. R. 1971. Evaluative research and community mental health. In A. E. Bergen and S. L. Garfield (eds.), *Handbook of psychotherapy and behavior change*. New York: Wiley.

Rutt, C. N., and Offord, D. R. 1971. Prenatal and perinatal complications in childhood schizophrenics and their siblings. *Journal of Nervous and Mental Disease* 152(5):324-331.

Rutter, M.; Tizard, J.; and Whitmore, K. (eds.). 1970. *Education, health and behavior*. London: Longmans.

Scarr-Salapatek, S. 1971. Race, social class and IQ. *Science* 114(4016).

SCAT (Cooperative School and College Ability Tests). 1966. Grades 10-12. Princeton, N.J.: Cooperative Tests and Services, Educational Testing Services.

Schachter, M. 1950. Observations on the prognosis of children born following trauma at birth. *American Journal of Mental Deficiency* 5:456-463.

Shepherd, M.; Oppenheim, B.; and Mitchell, S. 1971. *Childhood behavior and mental health*. New York: Grune & Stratton.

Sloggett, Barbara B.; Gallimore, Ronald; and Kubany, Edward S. 1970. A comparative analysis of fantasy need achievement among high and low achieving male Hawaiian-Americans. *Journal of Cross-Cultural Psychology* 1:53-61.

Smith, A. C.; Glick, G. L.; Ferris, G.; and Sellmann, A. 1972. Prediction of developmental outcome at seven years from prenatal, perinatal and postnatal events. *Child Development* 43:495-507.

Smith, R. G.; Steinhoff, P. G.; Diamond, M.; and Brown, N. 1971. Abortion in Hawaii: The first 124 days. *American Journal of Public Health* 61:530-542.

Sontag, L. W. 1971. The history of longitudinal research: Implications for the future. *Child Development* 42:987-1002.

Stabenau, J., and Pollin, W. 1969. Experiential differences for schizophrenics as compared with their non-schizophrenic siblings: Twin and family studies. In M. Roff and D. Ricks (eds.), *Life history research in psychopathology*. Minneapolis: University of Minnesota Press.

Stennett, R. G. 1966. Emotional handicap in the elementary years, phase or disease? *American Journal of Orthopsychiatry* 36:444-449.

STEP (Sequential Tests of Educational Progress). 1966. Grades 10-12. Princeton, N.J.: Cooperative Tests and Services, Educational Testing Services.

Stewart, Lawrence H.; Dole, Arthur A.; and Harris, Yeuell Y. 1967.

Cultural differences in abilities during high school. *American Educational Research Journal* 4:19–30.

Stewart, M.; Ferris, A.; Pitts, N., Jr.; and Craig, A. G. 1966. The hyperactive child syndrome. *American Journal of Orthopsychiatry* 36:861–867.

Stott, D. H. 1969. The congenital background in behavior disturbance. In M. Roff and D. Ricks (eds.), *Life history research in psychopathology*. Minneapolis: University of Minnesota Press.

Thomas, A.; Chess, G.; and Birch, H. 1968. *Temperament and behavior disorders in children*. New York: New York University Press.

Thurstone, L., and Thurstone, T. G. 1954. *SRA primary mental abilities: examiner's manual*. Chicago: Science Research Associates.

Tuft, L. T., and Goldfarb, W. 1964. Prenatal and perinatal factors in childhood schizophrenia. *Developmental Medicine and Child Neurology* 6:32–43.

Tulkien, S. R. 1972. An analysis of the concept of cultural deprivation. *Developmental Psychology* 6:326–339.

U.S. Joint Commission on the Mental Health of Children. 1970. *Crisis in child mental health: Challenge for the 1970's*. New York: Harper & Row.

Vorster, D. 1960. An investigation into the part played by organic factors in childhood schizophrenia. *Journal of Mental Science* 106:494–522.

Wechsler, David. 1949. *Wechsler intelligence scale for children*. New York: Psychological Corporation.

Weiss, G.; Minde, K.; Werry, J. S.; Douglas, V.; and Nemeth, E. 1971. Studies on the hyperactive child—VIII: Five-year follow-up. *Archives of General Psychiatry* 24:409–414.

Wender, P. H. 1971. *Minimal brain dysfunction in children*. New York: Wiley.

Werner, Emmy (ed.). 1967. *The teenage parent: Early marriage and childbearing*. 2nd ed. Mimeographed. University of California, Davis.

Werner, E.; Bierman, J.; and French, F. 1971. *The children of Kauai: A longitudinal study from the prenatal period to age ten*. Honolulu: University of Hawaii Press.

Werner, E.; Bierman, J. M.; French, F.; Simonian, K.; Connor, A.; Smith, R.; and Campbell, M. 1968. Reproductive and environmental casualties: A report on the 10 year follow-up of the children of the Kauai pregnancy study. *Pediatrics* 42:112–127.

Werner, E., and Gallistel, E. 1961. Prediction of outstanding performance, delinquency and emotional disturbance from childhood evaluation. *Child Development* 32:255–260.

Werner, E.; Honzik, M. P.; and Smith, R. S. 1968. Prediction of intelligence and achievement at 10 years from 20 months pediatric and psychologic examinations. *Child Development* 39:1063–1075.

Werner, E.; Simonian, K.; Bierman, J. M.; and French, F. 1967. Cumulative effect of perinatal complications and deprived environment on physical, intellectual and social development of preschool children. *Pediatrics* **39**:490–505.

Werner, E.; Simonian, K.; and Smith, R. S. 1967. Reading achievement, language functioning and perceptual-motor development of 10 and 11 year olds. *Perceptual and Motor Skills* **25**:409–420.

————. 1968. Ethnic and socioeconomic status differences in abilities and achievement among preschool and school-age children in Hawaii. *Journal of Social Psychology* **75**:43–59.

Werry, J.; Minde, K.; Guzman, A.; Weiss, G.; Dogan, K.; and Hoy, E. 1972. Studies on the hyperactive child—VII: Neurological status compared with neurotic and normal children. *American Journal of Orthopsychiatry* **4**(3):441–450.

Willerman, Lee. 1972. Biosocial influences on human development. *American Journal of Orthopsychiatry* **42**(3):452–462.

Zitrin, A.; Feuber, P.; and Cohen, D. 1964. Prenatal and paranatal factors in mental disorders of children. *Journal of Nervous and Mental Disease* **138**:357–361.

Index

About the Authors

Emmy E. Werner is professor of Human Development and Research Child Psychologist at the University of California, Davis. She has served as a consultant to various government agencies, including UNICEF and the Department of Health, Education, and Welfare, and is the recipient of the Elsie Worcester Memorial Award for Exceptional Accomplishment in the Area of Special Education. Dr. Werner is the contributor of some fifty articles to prominent professional journals and is the author (with Jessie M. Bierman and Fern E. French) of *The Children of Kauai.*

Ruth S. Smith is a clinical psychologist, presently in private practice on Kauai. Her experience includes clinical work at the University of Washington Child Guidance Clinic, the Merrill-Palmer School in Detroit, and with the State of Hawaii Division of Mental Health. Mrs. Smith was on the faculty of Bard College and has taught courses at the University of Hawaii and Kauai Community College. She has lived on Kauai for eighteen years and has co-authored, with Dr. Werner and others, several publications related to the earlier phases of the Kauai study.

⅄ *Production Notes*

The text of this book has been designed by Roger J. Eggers and typeset on the Unified Composing System by the design & production staff of The University Press of Hawaii.

The text and display typeface is English Times.

Offset presswork and binding is the work of The Maple Press Company. Text paper is Glatfelter P & S Offset, basis 55.

DATE DUE	
NOV 0 4 1996	

Library Store #47-0119 Peel Off Pressure Sensitive